中国器官移植发展报告
（2020）

黄洁夫　主编

中国器官移植发展基金会　组织编写

中国科学技术出版社
·北　京·

图书在版编目（CIP）数据

中国器官移植发展报告 . 2020 / 黄洁夫主编 . — 北京 : 中国科学技术出版社，2022.3

ISBN 978-7-5046-9293-1

Ⅰ . ①中… Ⅱ . ①黄… Ⅲ . ①器官移植—研究报告—中国— 2020 Ⅳ . ① R617

中国版本图书馆 CIP 数据核字 (2021) 第 222609 号

策划编辑	宗俊琳　焦健姿
责任编辑	孙　超
文字编辑	宗俊琳　史慧勤
装帧设计	佳木水轩
责任印制	李晓霖

出　　版	中国科学技术出版社
发　　行	中国科学技术出版社有限公司发行部
地　　址	北京市海淀区中关村南大街 16 号
邮　　编	100081
发行电话	010-62173865
传　　真	010-62179148
网　　址	http://www.cspbooks.com.cn

开　　本	710mm×1000mm　1/16
字　　数	213 千字
印　　张	9.25
版　　次	2022 年 3 月第 1 版
印　　次	2022 年 3 月第 1 次印刷
印　　刷	天津翔远印刷有限公司
书　　号	ISBN 978-7-5046-9293-1 / R·2802
定　　价	68.00 元

《中国器官移植发展报告（2020）》
编委会

前　言

　　器官移植是 20 世纪生命医学科学的一项重大进展，经过从临床试验到临床应用的发展过程，技术逐渐成熟，成为治疗终末期器官功能衰竭的有效医疗手段，拯救了众多的器官功能衰竭患者，促进了我国生命医学科学的发展。由于器官移植需要一个可供移植的器官，无论是公民逝世后捐献器官还是亲属捐献的活体器官，均涉及社会、宗教、伦理、政治、法治等深层次问题，因而器官移植与国家的传统文化和社会经济发展密切相关。

　　器官移植事业要遵循全世界公认的伦理准则，又要扎根本国的传统文化，立足于社会发展阶段的国情。我国政府高度重视发展人体器官捐献与移植事业，2006 年3 月 16 日，原国家卫生部印发《人体器官移植技术临床应用管理暂行规定》（卫医发〔2006〕94 号），明确器官移植管理要求，并出台了器官移植技术管理规范，对器官移植技术进行了准入管理。同年，全国人体器官移植临床应用管理峰会在广州召开，移植界医务人员凝聚共识，发表了《广州宣言》。2007 年 5 月，《人体器官移植条例》（以下简称《条例》）由国务院正式颁布实施，标志着我国人体器官捐献与移植工作体系建设走上法治化的轨道。同年，原国家卫生部发布《卫生部办公厅关于境外人员申请人体器官移植有关问题的通知》（卫办医发〔2007〕110 号），明确规定"禁止国外公民以旅游的名义到中国进行器官移植"。2010 年，原国家卫生部与中国红十字会总会共同启动了公民逝世后器官捐献试点工作，立足于中国社会发展阶段与传统文化基础，建立了中国红十字会作为第三方参与的人体器官捐献体系，并依据国际通行准则和中国国情，创新性地提出了公民逝世后自愿器官捐献三类标准：Ⅰ类，脑死亡后器官捐献；Ⅱ类，心脏死亡后器官捐献；Ⅲ类，脑 - 心双死亡后器官捐献。这为中国公民逝世后自愿器官捐献奠定了理论基础。2011 年，我国出台了《刑法修正案（八）》，增设"组织出卖人体器官罪"，将组织买卖人体器官作为严重的刑事犯罪予以严厉打击，进一步加强了器官捐献的法治化建设。2010 年，出台文件明确器官分配原则。2011 年，中国人体器官分配与共享计算机系统（COTRS）上线运行，通过计算机系统进行科学公平分配，并有序组建器官捐献协调员队伍。

　　2013 年 2 月 25 日，原国家卫生部与中国红十字会总结试点工作经验，正式在全国范围内开展公民逝世后自愿器官捐献工作。同年8月，原国家卫生和计划生育委员会出台了《人体捐献器官获取与分配管理规定（试行）》，组建OPO并划定服务范围，明确要求各移植医疗机构，严格使用COTRS实施器官分配，任何机构、组织和个人不得在器官分配系统外擅自分配捐献器官，确保人体捐献器官分配科学、公平，并实现移植器官可溯源管理。2013年12月19日，中共中央办公厅、国务院办公厅印发《关于党员干部带头推动殡葬改革的意见》，鼓励党员、干部去世后捐献器官或遗体。2014年3月，人体器官移植技术临床应用委员会（OTC）与人体器官捐献委员会合并成立了中国器官捐献与移植委员会，对器官移植事业进行顶层设计。十年磨一剑，我国逐步建立了人体器官捐献与移植体系，包括人体器官捐献体系、人体器官获取与分配体系、人体器官移植临床服务体系、人体器官获取与移植质控体系和人体器官捐献与移植监管体系，并在全社会大力弘扬器官捐献的大爱精神，公平、透明、阳光的公民自愿器官捐献的大气候正在全社会逐步形成。自2015年1月1日起，我国移植器官均来源于公民捐献，实现了器官来源的历史性改变。

健康是人类的共同追求，世界卫生与健康事业离不开中国持续不懈的努力，我国卫生与健康事业也需要其他国家的支持。近年来，我国逐步加强与各国的交流合作，全面展示了我国器官移植顶层设计、制度建设、法律法规及工作体系，并通过世界卫生组织全球器官捐献与移植监测网向国际社会提供有关数据及分析结果，公开透明地展示我国人体器官捐献与移植工作成果。我国的改革得到了国际社会的认可和支持，在 The Lancet、Transplantation 等国际器官移植权威期刊上共同发表了一系列推进改革的文章。国际器官移植领域的不少专家直接参与和见证了我国器官移植改革全进程，也十分认可我国器官移植改革所取得的进步。2016年8月，第26届世界器官移植协会年会在中国香港举行，这是首次在我国举行的世界器官移植大会，黄洁夫教授在大会开幕式上作了大会主旨演讲，向全世界介绍中国器官移植改革的十年历程。同年10月，在北京人民大会堂金色大厅召开了第一届中国－国际器官捐献大会，众多国际器官移植协会专家出席并共同见证了中国器官移植正式走向国际社会。2017年2月，中国受邀出席梵蒂冈教皇科学院举办的反对世界器官贩卖国际高峰论坛，我国参会代表实事求是地发出中国声音，讲好中国故事，并获得了高度认可。器官捐献与移植的"中国方案"被世界卫生组织誉为"中国对世界移植的创新和贡献"，正如世界卫生组织移植特别工作委员会主席弗兰克·德尔莫尼教授在梵蒂冈会议上讲到的，"你们的骨头也是我们的骨头，你们的进步也是我们的进步"。中国逐步融入了世界器官移植大家庭。世界卫生组织主管移植的官员约瑟·雷蒙·努涅斯教授指出，"世界器官移植像艘大船，中国以前不在船上，也不知道中国驶向何方，但从2015年后，中国已经站在了船的中央"。2018年3月，中国的器官移植改革经验在联合国与梵蒂冈教皇科学院共同举办的"践行伦理行动"会议上发表了最终会议宣言。会议上发布的"梵蒂冈教皇科学院践行伦理道德会议宣言"中提到，"中国模式的基本特征体现了中国政府持续改革的坚定决心，黄洁夫教授领导下的移植界专业人士与政府通力合作，高效落实了器官移植改革措施"。2018年5月，中国参加第七十一届世界卫生大会器官移植边会，我国100多名移植专家出席了会议并在大会上介绍了中国器官移植的改革经验。世界卫生组织总干事谭德赛博士称赞并感谢中国为世界移植做出的贡献。同年8月，由我国倡议建立的世界卫生组织器官捐献与移植特别工作委员会在西班牙马德里召开的第二十七届世界移植大会期间正式成立，该委员会由31名专家共同组成；黄洁夫被聘为世界卫生组织移植顾问，中国开始为世界移植全球治理工作贡献中国智慧。

近年来，我国相继颁布和建立了有利于器官捐献与移植的法律法规。例如，2016年国家交通、航空、铁路等六部门联合建立了器官转运绿色通道，为拯救生命赢得宝贵时间；2017年5月，《中华人民共和国红十字会法》修订，明确推动器官捐献的工作要求。至此，我国器官捐献和移植的数量和质量也得到了快速发展。2015—2018年，我国公民亲属间活体捐献数量保持稳定，每年为2200～2500例。器官捐献数量持续增加，2015年完成公民逝世后器官捐献2766例；2016年完成公民逝世后器官捐献4080例；2017年完成公民逝世后器官捐献5146例；2018年，公民逝世后器官捐献达6302例，实施器官移植手术20 201例，移植手术总量居世界第二位。自2019年起，我国器官捐献与移植工作由高速度增长转向高质量发展，坚持以供给侧结构性改革为主线，在积极推动捐献的同时，进一步优化器官移植临床服务体系布局，加强捐献、获取和分配管理力度，在质的大幅度提升中实现量的有效增长，努力实现更高质量、更有效率、更加公平、可持续的发展。2019年完成公民逝世后器官捐献5818例。2020年，尽管受到新冠肺炎疫情影响，仍实现公民逝世后器官捐献5222例。除了器官移植数量的发展之外，器官移植医疗质量也不断完善，1年和5年存活率已达到了世界先进水平。器官移植创新技术也在不断涌现，例如，自体肝移植、无缺血器官移植等器官移植技术实现国际领跑；供受者血型不相容肾脏移植技术得到突破；单中心儿童肝移植、心脏移植、肺脏移植临床服务能力居世界前列；

器官保存与供体器官维护技术不断改进；肝癌肝移植与乙肝肝移植临床经验已逐步得到国际认可等。经过多年不懈努力，我国人体器官捐献与移植事业取得快速发展，基本形成了科学公正、遵循伦理、符合我国国情和文化的人体器官捐献与移植工作模式，确定了人体器官捐献与移植工作的基本思路，形成了"政府主导、部门协作、行业推动、社会支持"的工作格局。

2019年10月，中国共产党十九届四中全会明确提出了坚持和完善中国特色社会主义制度、推进国家治理体系和治理能力现代化的要求。2020年5月28日《中华人民共和国民法典》正式颁布，在第四编"人格权"部分中明确提出"公民可自愿器官捐献"及"禁止器官买卖行为"。"打铁还需自身硬"，新的时代对器官移植提出了更高要求。我们将积极响应党的号召，推进器官移植改革的现代化进程，加强制度建设、体系建设与能力建设，不断完善自己，维护来之不易的改革成果。我们将通过不懈努力，建设一个完善的、符合伦理和世界卫生组织准则的人体器官捐献与移植工作体系，努力攀登器官移植学科相关科学技术高峰，积极推进"一带一路"器官捐献与移植国际合作，为建设"人类命运共同体"做出应有的贡献。

本报告记录了中国器官移植历史发展新阶段的成绩，将向世界展示中国器官移植改革经验与成果，中国器官移植发展基金会将每年组织编写出版，实现中英双语发布。

编　者

2021年8月

目　录

第1章 中国人体器官获取

一、中国人体器官获取组织发展历程

人体器官获取组织（Organ Procurement Organization，OPO）作为器官捐献和器官移植的基石和桥梁，是公民器官捐献时代的新生机构，是围绕人体捐献器官获取与分配管理诸多重要环节与流程开展管理与工作的专业队伍，由省级卫生健康行政部门遴选组建，专门从事公民逝世后人体器官捐献与获取工作的专业组织，由外科医师、神经内外科医师、重症医学科医师及护士、人体器官捐献协调员等组成，其主要职责包括器官捐献宣教，捐献者信息采集，潜在供体识别、评估、维护、转运，器官获取、保存、分配、运输，以及捐献后的善后、缅怀等工作。

2013年8月13日，原国家卫生和计划生育委员会出台《人体捐献器官获取与分配管理规定（试行）》（国卫医发〔2013〕11号），要求各省级卫生健康行政部门遴选组建OPO，明确划分OPO服务范围，并要求所有捐献器官必须通过中国人体器官分配与共享计算机系统（China Organ Transplant Response System，COTRS）实现公平、透明、可溯源的器官获取与分配。OPO在这一时期正式进入中国器官捐献与移植的历史舞台。

2013年9月3日原国家卫生和计划生育委员会下发了《关于加强人体捐献器官获取与分配管理工作的通知》（国卫医发〔2013〕16号），赋予了省级卫生健康行政部门规划辖区内OPO建设和管理的责权，对各地OPO服务区域的划分、建立、变更提供了指导意见。2014年3月20日，中国医院协会人体器官获取组织联盟宣告成立，标志着我国器官获取组织有了行业管理机构，为统一管理和行业自律奠定了基础。随后，在2014年12月3日召开的"2014年中国OPO联盟研讨会"上，中国人体器官捐献与移植委员会主任黄洁夫宣布自2015年1月1日起公民自愿器官捐献成为唯一合法器官来源，标志着中国器官移植事业进入历史发展新阶段。

2016 年 10 月 16 日，中国医院协会在原 OPO 联盟的基础上，重组成立中国医院协会器官获取与分配工作委员会（以下简称"工作委员会"），标志着我国 OPO 建设迈入了新的征程，工作委员会在国家卫生健康委员会医政医管局、中国人体器官捐献与移植委员会的监督和指导下，承接中国人体器官捐献与移植"五大工作体系"中的人体器官获取与分配体系建设工作。

受国家卫生健康委员会和中国人体器官捐献与移植委员会委托，工作委员会在前期工作的基础上，组织专家制订了多部行业规范，其中《人体器官获取与移植成本核算和经费管理试行办法（草案）》于 2017 年 1 月 1 日刊发，为全国 OPO 在建设过程中积极探索和逐步规范成本核算和经费管理提供了参考依据；《人体器官获取组织管理办法》被国家卫生健康委员会采纳，并在全国医政行政管理部门征求意见，经修订为《人体捐献器官获取与分配管理规定》（国卫医发〔2019〕2 号），由国家卫生健康委员会于 2019 年 1 月 17 日印发执行。2019 年 2 月，为规范 OPO 建设发展，建立完善人体器官获取组织质量管理与控制体系，国家卫生健康委员会办公厅印发《人体器官获取组织基本要求和质量控制指标》，该文件纳入并修订了由工作委员会起草的《人体器官获取组织（OPO）质量控制标准》，结合 OPO 发展现状，明确了人体器官获取组织所在医疗机构、人员及技术管理的基本要求，制订了人体器官获取组织的 9 项质量控制指标，对人体器官获取组织的规范管理发挥了重要作用。

二、OPO 机构分布

2020 年，全国共有 133 个 OPO。实行全省统一 OPO 管理的省份有山西、吉林、天津、海南；实行联合 OPO 管理的省份有广东、北京、湖南、上海、河北和福建（图 1-1）。

三、器官捐献情况

2020 年，公民逝世后器官捐献量前十位的省份依次为广东（818 例）、北京（496 例）、山东（390 例）、湖南（373 例）、广西（356 例）、河南（309 例）、浙江（280 例）、湖北（278 例）、江西（250 例）和陕西（202 例）。14 个省份 PMP 超过全国水平

（3.70），PMP 前十位的省份依次为北京（22.66）、广西（7.10）、广东（6.49）、海南（6.05）、湖南（5.61）、江西（5.53）、陕西（4.81）、湖北（4.81）、浙江（4.34）和上海（4.02）（图 1-2）。

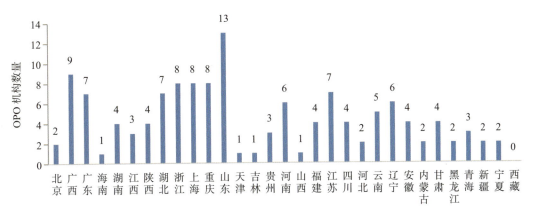

▲ 图 1-1　2020 年各省（区、市）OPO 的数量

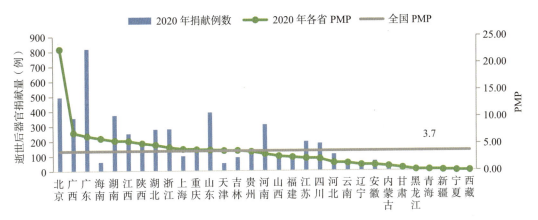

▲ 图 1-2　每百万人口器官捐献率

四、器官产出情况

2020 年，全国每位捐献者平均产出器官数 3.14 个，平均产出肝脏器官数 0.94 个、肾脏器官数 1.90 个、心脏器官数 0.11 个、肺脏器官数 0.18 个（图 1-3 至图 1-7）。

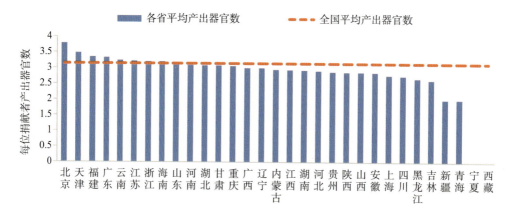

▲ 图 1-3　各省（区、市）每位捐献者产出器官数

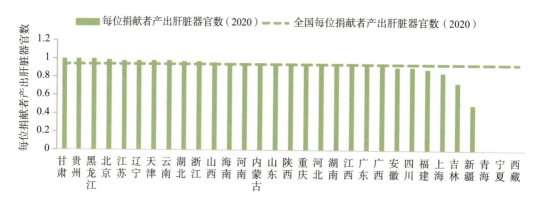

▲ 图 1-4　各省（区、市）每位捐献者产出肝脏器官数

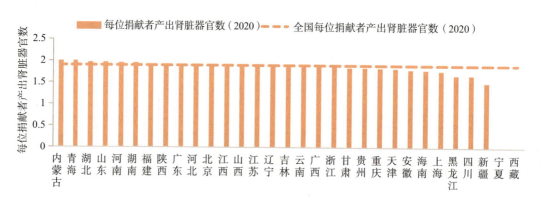

▲ 图 1-5　各省（区、市）每位捐献者产出肾脏器官数

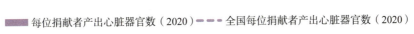
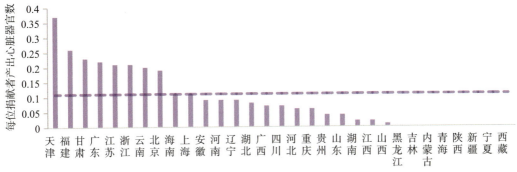

▲ 图 1-6　各省（区、市）每位捐献者产出心脏器官数

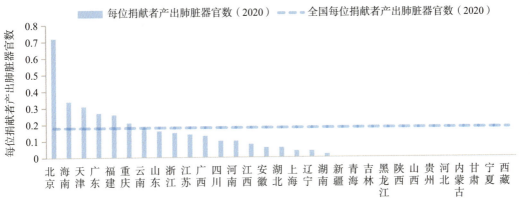

▲ 图 1-7　各省（区、市）每位捐献者产出肺脏器官数

在年器官捐献大于 20 例的 75 个 OPO 中，器官产出率前十位的 OPO 是北京南部联合体人体器官获取组织（4.21）、广州医科大学附属第一医院（4.07）、苏州大学附属第一医院（3.72）、北京北部联合体人体器官获取组织（3.71）、广州医科大学附属第二医院（3.7）、浙江大学医学院附属第二医院（3.6）、广东省人民医院（3.6）、青岛大学附属医院(3.47)、郑州市第七人民医院(3.46)、天津市第一中心医院(3.46)。

五、捐献器官获取质量控制内容

捐献器官获取质量控制包括 OPO 机构、器官捐献者和捐献器官质量控制三个层面。

1. OPO 机构质量控制

在 OPO 机构层面，从规范、绩效、技术三个方面，加强 OPO 机构的质量控制。制定 OPO 质量控制与管理指标 29 项，其中包括核心指标 9 项、绩效指标 9 项、技术指标 6 项、参考指标 5 项。经国家卫生健康委员会印发质量控制指标 9 项，即器官捐献转化率、器官捐献分类占比、平均器官产出率、获取器官利用率、边缘器官比率、器官病理检查率、器官保存液细菌培养阳性率、移植器官原发性无功能发生率、移植器官术后功能延迟性恢复发生率。

2. 器官捐献者质量控制

对器官捐献者的质量控制工作内容包括病史情况、临床评估、血管活性药物用量、实验室检查结果、肿瘤筛查、感染筛查、器官穿刺病理评估，为移植医疗机构提供质量控制服务。

3. 捐献器官质量控制

对获取后的捐献器官的质量控制工作内容包括供肝、供肾、供心、供肺、供胰等进行形态、解剖、损伤等评估。

六、特点与展望

在党中央、国务院支持下，在国家卫生健康委员会和中国红十字会总会的直接领导下，中国人体器官捐献与移植委员会带领业界人士齐心协力，经过十余年实践摸索，在严格遵循国际公认的伦理学原则的基础上，创建了符合中国国情的器官捐献与移植的"中国模式"，成功实现器官来源的转型，确保捐献器官公正分配和可溯源性，充分保障器官捐献者和移植受者的权益。为进一步巩固我国器官捐献与移植事业的健康有序发展，建立和健全符合中国模式的 OPO 是关键一环。为进一步推进器官获取工作，需重点做好以下几个方面。

1. 规范 OPO 管理

规范 OPO 组织架构、人员结构、工作职能、操作流程，并进行有效的过程控制和监督管理，是提升 OPO 质量的必要条件。根据国家卫生健康委员会《人体器官获取与分配管理规定》（国卫医发〔2019〕2 号），在现有基础上结合中国国情，按照省级卫生健康行政部门规划，在满足各地医疗需要的前提下合理设置、逐步统一 OPO，保障 OPO 在划定的区域内规范开展器官捐献与获取工作，应为下一步的重点发展方向。

2. 规范 OPO 绩效评价与质量控制

中国公民逝世后自愿器官捐献促进了我国器官移植事业向法制化、伦理化、国际同步化发展，同时也促进了中国器官获取组织的派生与建设。中国公民逝世后自愿器官捐献的健康发展有赖于 OPO 体系建设，包括供体甄别、死亡判定、捐献者维护器官、质量优化、质量评估以及器官获取技术研究及规范，这些体系的完善与捐献者、器官质量密切相关。因此，亟须制订捐献者与器官质量控制标准，严格把控捐献者与器官质量，为终末期器官衰竭患者提供优质的医疗服务。

3. 建立器官获取与分配的互信机制

通过加强 OPO 关于供体评估、器官质量评估、感染、病理等指标的填报，规范和完善数据共享，提升 OPO 与移植医院之间的器官分配互信度，减少捐献器官弃用及损失，挽救更多器官功能衰竭患者。

4. 建立 OPO 经费管理机制

以省域为单位制订捐献器官获取收费标准，推进 OPO 运行费用规范管理，建立完善、统一、合理的公民逝世后捐献器官获取、修复、维护、保存、运送、检验、分配及移植等收费标准，将器官获取成本阳光、透明地计入器官移植费用，促进人体器官获取工作健康发展。

第 2 章 中国人体器官分配与共享

本章内容为基于中国人体器官分配与共享计算机系统（China Organ Transplant Response System，COTRS）的数据分析，统计范围是中国内地，不包含港澳台地区。

自 2015 年 1 月 1 日至 2020 年 12 月 31 日，中国公民逝世后器官捐献（deceased donation，DD）累计完成 29 334 例。2020 年，中国完成公民逝世后器官捐献 5222 例，器官移植手术 17 897 例。每百万人口器官捐献率（per million population，PMP）从 2015 年的 2.01 上升至 2020 年的 3.70。

中国人体器官捐献和移植的五大工作体系包括人体器官捐献体系、人体器官获取与分配体系、人体器官移植临床服务体系、人体器官获取与移植质控体系和人体器官捐献与移植监管体系（图 2-1）。目前，中国已实现了科学、公平、公正的器官分配。

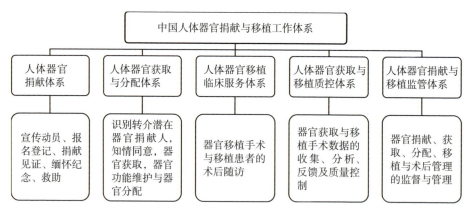

▲ 图 2-1 中国人体器官捐献与移植工作体系（不包含港澳台地区）

COTRS 是《人体器官移植条例》第六条、第二十二条和《刑法修正案（八）》第二百三十四条等有关器官移植和捐献法律条款的重要体现和落实。2018 年，国家卫生健康委员会印发了《关于印发中国人体器官分配与共享基本原则和核心政策的通知》（国卫医发〔2018〕24 号），对《卫生部关于印发中国人体器官分配与共享基本原则和肝脏与肾脏移植核心政策的通知》（卫医管发〔2010〕113 号）进行了修订，并制订了心脏、肺脏分配与共享核心政策，形成了《中国人体器官分配与共享基本原则和核心政策》（以下简称"器官分配核心政策"）。

我国器官分配核心政策依据国务院颁布的《人体器官移植条例》规定的原则和标准建立，符合世界卫生组织要求的国际准则，同时也具有我国的特色。例如，我国为了鼓励公民逝世后器官捐献，对于在同一地理分配层级内符合公民逝世后器官捐献者的直系亲属、配偶、三代以内旁系血亲或登记成为中国人体器官捐献志愿者 3 年以上的，在排序时将获得优先权，同时活体器官捐献者在需要进行器官移植手术治疗的，在排序时亦获得优先。

COTRS 是我国器官捐献与移植工作体系的重要组成部分，由"潜在器官捐献者识别系统""人体器官捐献人登记及器官匹配系统""人体器官移植等待者预约名单系统"三个子系统及监管平台组成。

作为执行我国器官分配与共享相关法律法规和科学政策的高度专用的关键系统，COTRS 执行国家器官科学分配政策，实施自动器官分配和共享，并向国家和地方监管机构提供全程监控，建立器官获取和分配的溯源性，最大限度地排除人为干预，保障器官分配的公平、公正、公开，是我国公民逝世后器官捐献工作赢得人民群众信任的重要基石。目前，COTRS 系统由中国器官移植发展基金会管理。

一、器官捐献与移植医疗资源分布

1. 全国器官获取组织分布

我国人体器官捐献与移植体系中，器官获取组织（Organ Procurement Organization，OPO）是依托医疗机构设立的器官捐献与获取专业团队。该团队由医务人员、器官捐献协调员、行政管理人员等组成。这一点与美国的 OPO 和西班牙的国家器官移植组织（Organization National De Transplant，ONT）有所不同。

截至 2020 年 12 月 31 日，全国共有 133 个 OPO（不包括香港、澳门特别行政区及台湾地区）。

2. 全国移植中心分布

截至 2020 年 12 月 31 日，除港澳台地区外，全国有 170 所具备器官移植资质的医疗机构，各省（区、市）移植医疗机构分布见图 2-2。其中，数量排名居前十位的省（区、市）为广东（19 所）、北京（17 所）、山东（12 所）、上海（11 所）、湖南（9 所）、浙江（9 所）、福建（8 所）、湖北（7 所）、广西（6 所）、河南（6 所）和辽宁（6 所）。

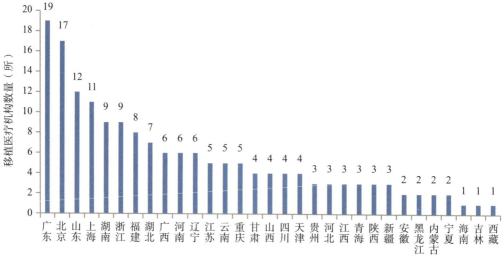

▲ 图 2-2　2020 年中国移植医疗机构分布情况（不包含港澳台地区）

二、人体器官捐献情况

1. 人体器官捐献情况

2015—2020 年，各年度中国公民逝世后器官捐献量分别为 2766 例、4080 例、5146 例、6302 例、5818 例和 5222 例，PMP 分别为 2.01、2.98、3.72、4.53、4.16 和 3.70（图 2-3）。

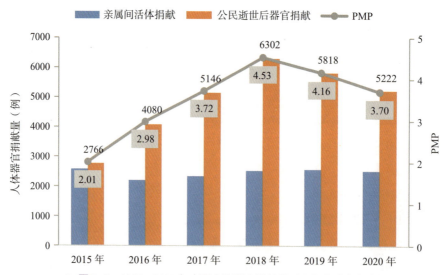

▲ 图 2-3　2015—2020 年中国人体器官捐献量（不包含港澳台地区）

2015—2019 年人口数来自《中国卫生健康统计年鉴》，2020 年人口数来源于国家统计局

　　2020 年，在全球新冠肺炎疫情席卷的严峻形势下，我国器官捐献与移植从业者为了救治终末期器官衰竭患者迎难而上、砥砺前行，随着 2020 年 4 月以来我国新冠肺炎疫情缓解，器官捐献工作快速恢复，2020 年 6 月起公民逝世后器官捐献量已恢复至 2019 年同期水平（图 2-4）。

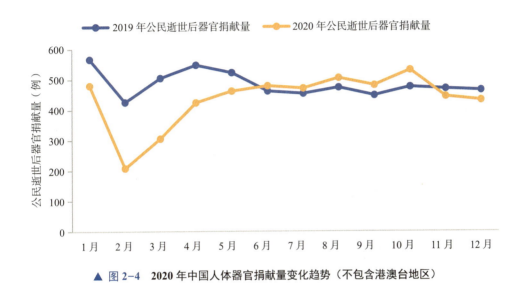

▲ 图 2-4　**2020 年中国人体器官捐献量变化趋势（不包含港澳台地区）**

　　2. 器官捐献者特征

　　2020 年，中国公民逝世后捐献者年龄中位数为 47 岁，儿童捐献者（18 岁以下）共 413 例，占 7.91%，其中 < 2 岁捐献者 81 例（19.61%），2—6 岁捐献者 99 例（23.97%），7—13 岁捐献者 117 例（28.33%），14—17 岁捐献者 116 例（28.09%）。捐献者性别以男性为主，占比为 80.89%。捐献者的血型以 O 型为主，占 37.03%；其次是 A 型和 B 型，分别占 27.75% 和 27.08%；AB 型占 8.14%（图 2-5）。44.33% 为中国Ⅰ类（脑死亡器官捐献），39.26% 为中国Ⅱ类（心死亡器官捐献），16.41% 为中国Ⅲ类（脑 - 心双死亡器官捐献）（图 2-6）。

　　2015—2020 年，创伤和脑血管意外为逝世后器官捐献者两大主要死亡原因，占所有死亡原因的 86.98%（图 2-7）。其中，脑血管意外死亡的捐献者占比逐年上升。2019 年起，脑血管意外超过创伤，成为中国公民逝世后器官捐献的主要死亡原因（图 2-8）。

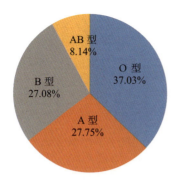

▲ 图 2-5 2020 年中国公民逝世后器官捐献者血型分布（不包含港澳台地区）

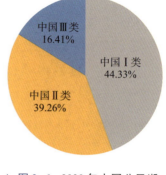

▲ 图 2-6 2020 年中国公民逝世后器官捐献者中国分类（不包含港澳台地区）

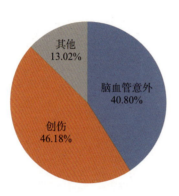

▲ 图 2-7 2015—2020 年逝世后器官捐献者死亡原因（不包含港澳台地区）

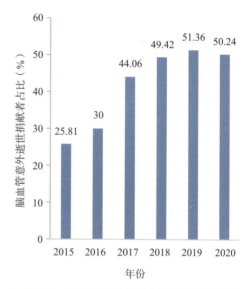

▲ 图 2-8 2015—2020 年脑血管意外逝世捐献者占比（不包含港澳台地区）

三、移植等待者情况

2015—2020 年，肝肾器官移植等待者数量（图 2-9）逐年增加。2020 年共有移植等待者 96 550 人活跃在等待名单中，包括肾脏移植等待者 78 324 人、肝脏移植等待者 15 991 人、心脏移植等待者 1423 人、肺脏移植等待者 812 人。同期，全国共有 17 897 人（18.54%）接受器官移植手术。

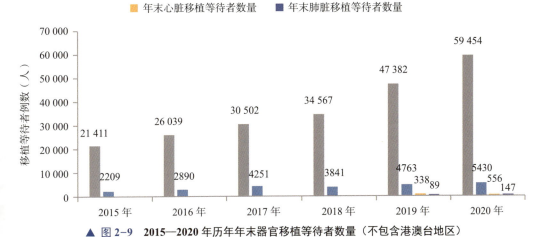

▲ 图 2-9　**2015—2020 年历年年末器官移植等待者数量（不包含港澳台地区）**

2020 年年末，全国仍有 59 454 人等待肾脏移植、5430 人等待肝脏移植。心脏、肺脏分配系统于 2018 年 10 月 22 日启用，2020 年年末仍有 556 人等待心脏移植，147 人等待肺脏移植。

除港澳台地区外，2020 年全国各省（区、市）肾脏移植等待者数量分布见图 2-10，其中排名前十位的省（区、市）依次为广东（7630 人）、浙江（5875 人）、湖南（5682 人）、四川（4949 人）、上海（4318 人）、湖北（4141 人）、河南（3041 人）、天津（2788 人）、山东（2609 人）和广西（2376 人）。

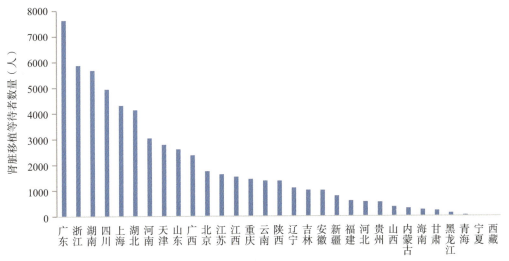

▲ 图 2-10　**2020 年年末中国肾脏移植等待者数量（不包含港澳台地区）**

2020 年年末，除港澳台地区外，全国各省（区、市）肝脏移植等待者数量分布见图 2-11，其中排名前十位的省（区、市）依次为四川（1240 人）、广东（810 人）、天津（656 人）、上海（411 人）、浙江（365 人）、北京（296 人）、湖北（256 人）、湖南（227 人）、江苏（154 人）和云南（150 人）。

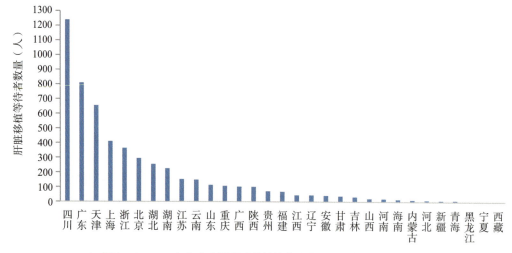

▲ 图 2-11　2020 年年末中国肝脏移植等待者数量（不包含港澳台地区）

2020 年年末，除港澳台地区外，全国各省（区、市）心脏移植等待者数量分布见图 2-12，其中排名前十位的省（区、市）依次为北京（154 人）、广东（69 人）、上海（60 人）、湖北（53 人）、河南（33 人）、浙江（33 人）、山东（30 人）、湖南（27人）、江苏（25 人）和天津（14 人）。

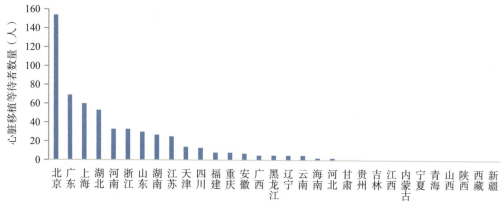

▲ 图 2-12　2020 年年末中国心脏移植等待者数量（不包含港澳台地区）

2020 年年末，除港澳台地区外，全国各省（区、市）肺脏移植等待者数量分布见图 2-13，其中排名前十位的省（区、市）依次为江苏（29 人）、广东（28 人）、浙江（25 人）、河南（11 人）、湖北（10 人）、安徽（9 人）、四川（9 人）、北京（8 人）、上海（8 人）和湖南（5 人）。

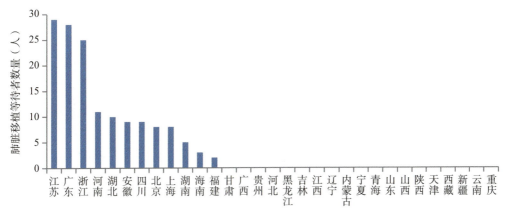

▲ 图 2-13　2020 年年末中国肺脏移植等待者数量（不包含港澳台地区）

四、器官利用情况

1. 逝世后器官捐献者产出器官情况

2015—2020 年，每位逝世后捐献者平均产出的肾脏器官数依次为 1.92 个、1.87 个、1.89 个、1.91 个、1.89 个和 1.90 个，平均年产出的肝脏器官数分别为 0.88 个、0.87 个、0.90 个、0.91 个、0.93 个和 0.94 个（图 2-14）。2020 年，每位捐献者平均产出的心脏器官数为 0.11 个，平均年产出的肺脏器官数为 0.18 个。2018 年，心脏、肺脏器官分配核心政策的制定以来，心脏、肺脏产出数量逐年上升，对比 2019 年，2020 年肺脏平均产出数量增加 20%。

2. 器官分配核心政策修订前后儿童肾脏移植对比

2018 年国家卫生健康委员会修订的器官分配核心政策，进一步全面推进和贯彻"十三五"时期优先保障儿童利益、推动公共资源优先向儿童配置的原则，结合肾脏疾病和透析治疗对少年儿童生长发育带来的严重的不良影响，18 岁以下捐献者的肾脏在全国范围内优先分配给 18 岁以下肾脏移植等待者，增加了儿童肾脏移植等待者获得移植的可能性。

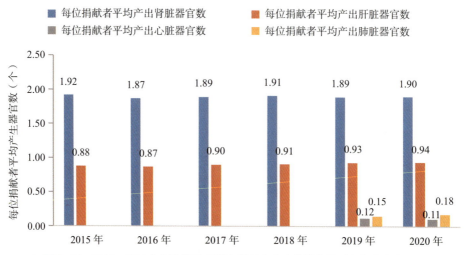

■ 每位捐献者平均产出肾脏器官数　　　■ 每位捐献者平均产出肝脏器官数
■ 每位捐献者平均产出心脏器官数　　　■ 每位捐献者平均产出肺脏器官数

▲ 图 2-14　2015—2020 年每位逝世后器官捐献者产出的器官数（不包含港澳台地区）

比较器官分配核心政策修订前后儿童肾脏移植情况显示，政策实施后，肾脏移植等待者中获得器官分配的儿童比例由 2% 上升至 3%，增幅为 50%。

3.绿色通道政策实施前后器官共享对比

原国家卫生和计划生育委员会、国家公安部、国家交通运输部、中国民用航空局、原中国铁路总公司和中国红十字会总会于 2016 年 5 月 6 日联合印发了《关于建立人体捐献器官转运绿色通道的通知》（以下简称《通知》），建立人体捐献器官转运绿色通道。通知明确了各方职责，目的是确保人体捐献器官转运流程的通畅，将器官转运环节对器官移植患者的质量安全影响减少到最低程度。

《通知》将器官转运分为一般流程及应急流程，转运过程中根据实际情况启动不同流程，实现人体捐献器官转运的快速通关与优先承运，提高转运效率，保障转运安全，减少因运输原因造成的器官浪费。

比较人体捐献器官转运绿色通道政策实施前后全国人体器官共享情况，结果显示，政策实施后，器官全国共享比例上升 5.8%，其中肾脏全国共享比例上升了 5.9%，肝脏全国共享比例上升了 3.9%（表 2-1）。

五、特点与展望

器官移植是人类医学发展的巨大成就，挽救了无数终末期疾病患者的生命。

表 2–1 绿色通道政策实施前后全国肝肾器官共享率（%）（不包含港澳台地区）

时间段	总体共享率（%）			肾脏共享率（%）			肝脏共享率（%）		
	政策前	政策后	变化	政策前	政策后	变化	政策前	政策后	变化
中心自用	75.0	67.4	−7.6	84.6	75.9	−8.7	53.2	49.9	−3.3
省内共享	12.6	14.4	**1.8**	10.5	13.3	**2.8**	17.3	16.7	−0.6
全国共享	12.4	18.2	**5.8**	4.9	10.8	**5.9**	29.5	33.4	**3.9**

2020 年中国器官捐献、移植数量均位居世界第二位。COTRS 作为我国器官分配与共享相关法律法规和科学政策的高度专用的关键系统，执行国家器官科学分配政策，保障器官分配的公平、公正、公开，发挥了重要的作用，还需注意以下几点。

1. 完善器官分配政策科学决策机制

器官分配的质量决定了器官和受者的生物匹配度，器官分配与共享的效率决定着器官的质量和器官利用效率，直接影响着移植受者的术后生存率和生活质量，科学合理的器官分配政策是关键。下一步，国家将成立"人体器官分配与共享计算机系统科学委员会"，由行业管理者和移植专家组成，建立健全定期工作机制，加强器官分配科学政策的研究，聚焦提升器官匹配质量、改善器官分配效率、降低移植等待者死亡率等方面的研究，研究并推动胰腺、小肠等器官分配政策，定期为政府提供决策依据。

2. 加强信息反馈，促进器官分配质量持续改进

经过 10 余年的努力，我国已经逐步构建了公平、公正、公开的人体器官捐献与分配体系，形成了"以信息化为手段，政府主导、行业自治、医院自查"的器官分配监督管理机制。同时建立了以大数据为支撑的信息化监管平台，实现了从器官捐献、获取、分配到移植的全过程可溯源管理。

应加强器官分配质量的动态监测，持续向器官获取组织、医疗机构、卫生健康主管部门反馈器官分配质量相关指标改善情况，提高不同医疗机构间器官分配质量同质化程度，缩小质量差异，提供更加高效科学的器官分配。

第3章 中国肝脏移植

本章内容主要基于中国肝脏移植注册系统（China Liver Transplant Registry，CLTR）的数据分析，统计范围是中国内地，不包含港澳台地区。

CLTR 是由国家卫生健康委员会建立的国家肝脏移植注册系统，要求全国具有肝脏移植资质的医疗机构必须及时、完整地向其填报移植相关信息。CLTR 通过对中国内地的肝脏移植情况进行动态、科学地分析，描述肝脏移植专业医疗质量现状，为国家监管部门制定移植相关的政策、法规提供了依据，为各移植中心提供了肝脏移植受者的科学管理工具。迄今为止，CLTR 已成为中国器官移植领域最重要的信息化系统以及肝脏移植学术交流平台之一。

一、肝脏移植医疗机构分布

截至 2020 年 12 月 31 日，全国共有 103 所具有肝脏移植资质的医疗机构。其中，肝脏移植医疗机构数量前十位的省（区、市）为北京（12 所）、广东（12 所）、上海（9 所）、山东（8 所）、浙江（6 所）、福建（5 所）、广西（5 所）、湖北（5 所）、湖南（4 所）、重庆（4 所）（图 3-1）。

2015—2020 年全国共实施肝脏移植 29 732 例，包括 25 584 例公民逝世后器官捐献肝脏移植（deceased donor liver transplantation，DDLT），占比 86.0%；4148 例亲属间活体肝脏移植（living-related donor liver transplantation，LDLT），占比 14.0%（图 3-2）。成人肝脏移植 24 423 例，占比 82.1%；儿童肝脏移植 5309 例，占比 17.9%。

2020 年，全国共实施肝脏移植手术 5842 例，包括 4954 例 DDLT，占比 84.8%；888 例 LDLT（包括 14 例多米诺肝脏移植，5 例废弃肝再利用），占比 15.2%。成人肝脏移植 4663 例，占比 79.8%；儿童肝脏移植 1179 例，占比 20.2%。2020 年实施肝脏移植例数排名前十位的省（区、市）依次为上海（1172 例）、浙江（810 例）、广东（684 例）、北京（556 例）、湖南（270 例）、天津（245 例）、河南（220 例）、江苏（197 例）、山东（194 例）、江西（180 例）。2020 年实施 100 例以上肝脏移植的省（区、市）有 16 个，移植总量占全国当年总例数的 92.4%（图 3-3）。宁夏、青海在 2020 年度未开展肝脏移植（西藏暂无具备肝脏移植资质的医疗机构）。

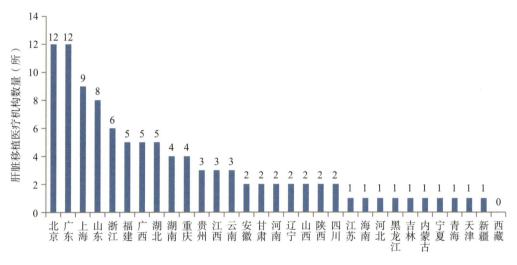

▲ 图 3-1　2020 年中国具有肝脏移植资质的医疗机构分布（不包含港澳台地区）

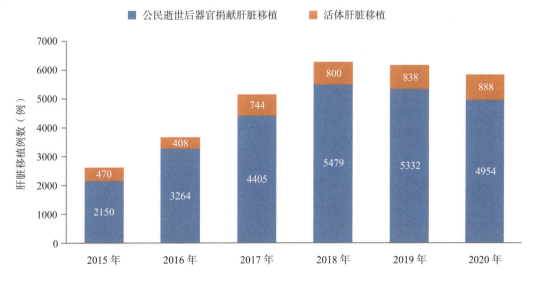

▲ 图 3-2　2015—2020 年中国肝脏移植例数（不包含港澳台地区）

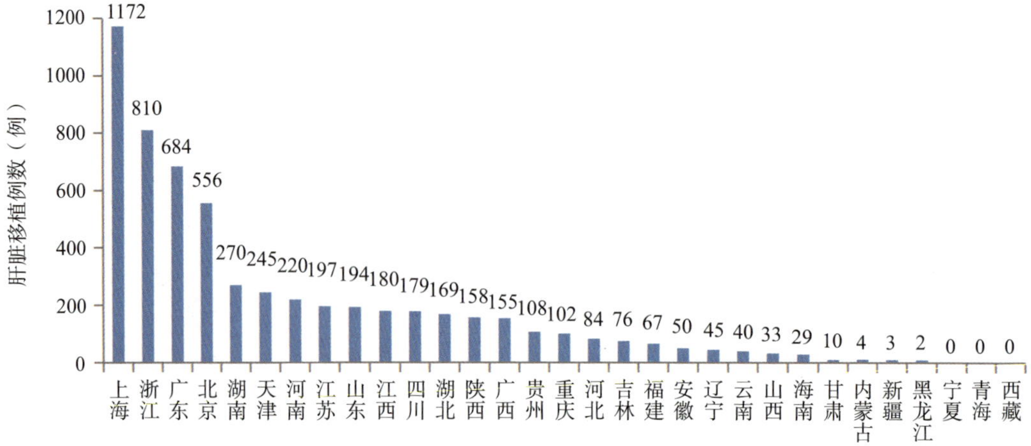

▲ 图 3-3　2020 年中国肝脏移植例数地区分布（不包含港澳台地区）

　　2020 年有 12 所医疗机构实施的肝脏移植例数在 150 例及以上，其移植总量占全国当年总例数的 52.6%（表 3-1）。

表 3-1　2020 年中国肝脏移植例数排名前 12 位的医疗机构（不包含港澳台地区）		
地　区	肝脏移植医疗机构	例　数
上海	上海交通大学医学院附属仁济医院	631
浙江	浙江大学医学院附属第一医院	432
上海	复旦大学附属中山医院	256
浙江	树兰（杭州）医院	255
天津	天津市第一中心医院	245
上海	复旦大学附属华山医院	228
广东	中山大学附属第三医院	218
北京	首都医科大学附属北京佑安医院	171
广东	中山大学附属第一医院	163
河南	郑州大学第一附属医院	161
北京	清华大学附属北京清华长庚医院	160
陕西	西安交通大学医学院第一附属医院	154

二、肝脏移植受者人口特征

2020 年我国肝脏移植受者的年龄均值 41.0 岁，中位数 48.1 岁；受者体重指数（body mass index，BMI）均值 22.1kg/m²，中位数 22.2kg/m²；以男性受者为主，占比 74.6%；受者血型以 O 型、A 型、B 型为主，且三种血型的受者各占 30% 左右，血型为 AB 型的受者占比最少（表 3-2）。儿童肝脏移植受者的年龄均值 2.6 岁，1 岁以下的肝脏移植受者有 689 例（11.8%），1—7 岁（不包含 7 岁）的有 333 例（5.7%），7—12 岁（不包含 12 岁）的有 95 例（1.6%），12—18 岁以下的有 62 例（1.1%）。

表 3-2　2020 年中国肝脏移植受者人口特征（不包含港澳台地区）		
变　量	均值 ± 标准差	占比（%）
年龄（岁）	41.0±21.5	—
BMI（kg/m²）	22.1±4.5	—
性别		
男	—	74.6
女	—	25.4
血型		
O 型	—	30.8
A 型	—	29.7
B 型	—	29.1
AB 型	—	10.4

三、肝脏移植质量安全分析

1. 肝脏移植重要临床指标

2020 年，我国 LDLT 的平均冷缺血时间、平均无肝期、术中平均失血量、术中平均输红细胞（red blood cell，RBC）量均低于 DDLT，LDLT 的平均手术时间略高于 DDLT（图 3-4 至图 3-8）。

2. 肝脏移植前后受者总胆红素的变化情况

分别对 2020 年 DDLT 受者和 LDLT 受者术前、术后各时间点的总胆红素变化情况进行分析，移植受者术后总胆红素平均值呈明显下降趋势（表 3-3）。

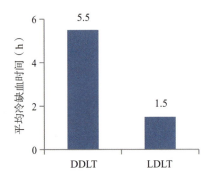

▲ 图 3-4　2020 年肝脏移植平均冷缺血时间（不包含港澳台地区）

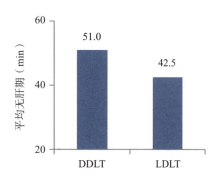

▲ 图 3-5　2020 年肝脏移植平均无肝期（不包含港澳台地区）

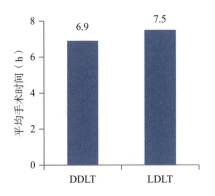

▲ 图 3-6　2020 年肝脏移植平均手术时间（不包含港澳台地区）

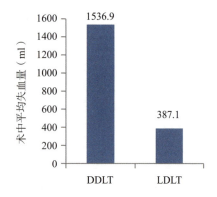

▲ 图 3-7　2020 年肝脏移植术中平均失血量（不包含港澳台地区）

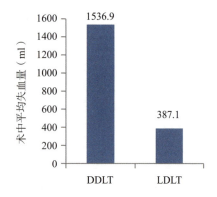

▲ 图 3-8　2020 年肝脏移植术中平均输红细胞（RBC）量（不包含港澳台地区）

表 3-3　2020 年肝脏移植受者术前、术后的总胆红素平均值（不包含港澳台地区）		
时　间	总胆红素平均值（μmol/L）	
	DDLT	LDLT
术前	242.4	223.0
术后 1 周	65.0	47.2
术后 2 周	46.9	26.5
术后 1 个月	31.8	16.6
术后 3 个月	19.3	9.9
术后 6 个月	20.0	10.8

3. 肝脏移植受者术后情况

(1) 术后 30 天内并发症：2020 年，我国 DDLT 受者术后 30 天内并发症发生率为 32.7%，主要为胸腔积液（20.6%）、术后感染（13.8%）、腹腔内积液 / 脓肿（12.6%）；LDLT 受者术后 30 天内并发症发生率为 19.4%，主要为术后感染（8.6%）、胸腔积液（5.4%）、血管并发症（5.3%）。

(2) 术后 30 天内死亡率：2020 年，我国 DDLT 受者术后 30 天内死亡率为 5.7%；LDLT 受者术后 30 天内死亡率为 3.4%。

(3) 肝脏移植术后受者、移植物生存情况：选取 2015—2020 年期间全国范围内开展的肝脏移植病例进行受者和移植物的生存分析，结果如下。

我国 DDLT 受者术后 1 年、3 年累计生存率分别为 83.6%、74.9%；LDLT 受者术后 1 年、3 年累计生存率分别为 91.8%、88.7%。

我国 DDLT 移植物术后 1 年、3 年累计生存率分别为 82.9%、73.8%；LDLT 移植物术后 1 年、3 年累计生存率分别为 91.1%、87.6%（表 3-4）。

表 3-4　2015—2020 年中国肝脏移植受者 / 移植物术后生存率（不包含港澳台地区）

分组	术后 1 年生存率（%）		术后 3 年生存率（%）	
	受者	移植物	受者	移植物
DDLT	83.6	82.9	74.9	73.8
LDLT	91.8	91.1	88.7	87.6

(4) 肝癌肝脏移植受者术后无瘤生存情况：2015—2020 年，我国肝癌肝脏移植受者术后 1 年和 3 年无瘤生存率分别为 77.2% 和 63.1%。

四、特点与展望

1. 儿童肝脏移植发展迅速

2020 年中国儿童肝脏移植 1179 例，占当年移植总量的 20.2%，较 2019 年儿童肝脏移植例数（1095 例）增加了 7.7%。其中，活体来源儿童肝脏移植 816 例；在 363 例儿童 DDLT 中，全肝肝脏移植占比 42.7%，减体积肝脏移植占比 3.0%，劈离式肝脏移植占比 54.3%。我国儿童肝脏移植最常见的适应证为先天性胆道闭锁，占 72.3%。

2. 亲属间活体肝脏移植占比较高

2020 年，我国亲属间活体肝脏移植占比为 15.2%，达到 888 例。在我国儿童肝脏移植中，亲属间活体来源占 69.2%，这反映出我国亲属间更加紧密的关系纽带。我国儿童 LDLT 中，移植肝类型前三位分别是左肝外侧叶（78.2%）、扩大的左肝外侧叶（8.6%）和左半肝（不含肝中静脉，5.0%）。

3. 原发病是肝癌的肝脏移植比例较高

我国是肝癌高发国家，2020 年的 DDLT 受者中，恶性肿瘤比例为 41.5%。我国提出的肝癌肝脏移植杭州标准得到了学术界的广泛认可和临床应用，可在扩大肝癌肝脏移植受者入选范围的同时，保持其生存率与国际水平无明显差异。

4. 不断探索肝脏移植手术方式和技术的创新

部分中心开展肝脏移植血管吻合技术的变革，吻合部位从胃十二指肠动脉改为脾动脉，显著改善术后肝脏血流，降低胆道并发症等发生率；开展无缺血肝脏移植；实施两人互换部分肝脏交叉辅助多米诺肝脏移植手术，为两个患有不同遗传代谢缺陷肝病的患者互换半个肝脏，实现了不需要器官捐献的器官移植等。

5. 建立并落实肝脏移植医疗质量管理与控制有关规范和制度

进一步完善捐献肝脏质量维护与评估体系，提高捐献肝脏质量，降低并发症发生率，提高受者生存率；加强术后重要并发症的监测，如术后早期肝功能不全、急性肾损伤、新发糖尿病等质控指标，以更加科学化、精细化的质控体系，实现全国肝脏移植临床质量、服务和疗效的提升。

6. 科学监管肝脏移植数据，挖掘有价值的信息

加强信息化建设，利用大数据思维和精细化管理开展临床研究，利用循证医学证据指导临床决策；汇聚临床优势资源，创新引领肝脏移植领域多中心高质量的临床研究，推进科研成果临床转化与应用，推动肝脏移植学科发展。

7. 新冠肺炎疫情的挑战

近年来，中国肝脏移植的数量和质量稳步提升，跻身国际前列。2020 年年初因新型冠状病毒肺炎疫情影响，1—5 月全国肝脏移植例数相较于 2019 年同期有所下降，6 月开始已超过 2019 年的同期水平。据不完全统计，我国有 3 例肝脏移植受者术后感染新冠肺炎，肝脏移植受者新冠肺炎的治疗，对于移植医院来说，无疑是一项重大挑战。3 例肝脏移植受者，经定点医院治疗后 COVID-19 咽拭子核酸检测均转阴性。

8. 劈离式肝脏移植前景

2020 年，DDLT 中有 387 例受者接受劈离式肝脏移植（split liver transplantation，SLT），SLT 的推行可以有效扩大供肝来源、减少患者移植等待时间，尤其是解决儿童器官短缺的问题，在 387 例 SLT 中，有超过 50% 的受者是儿童。我国劈离式肝脏移植中，移植肝类型前三位分别是左肝外侧叶（26.9%）、右半肝 + 第Ⅳ段（22.0%）、右半肝（包含肝中静脉，19.1%）。适合劈离的供肝及可接收 SLT 的受者选择标准还需进一步明确，以实现肝脏的最优化分配和安全应用。

第4章 中国肾脏移植

本章内容主要基于中国肾脏移植科学登记系统（Chinese Scientific Registry of Kidney Transplantation，CSRKT）数据分析，统计范围是中国内地，不包含港澳台地区。

CSRKT 是由国家卫生健康委员会建立的国家肾脏移植注册系统，要求全国具有肾脏移植资质的医疗机构必须及时、完整地向其填报移植相关信息。CSRKT 作为中国唯一的肾脏移植受者科学登记系统，通过对中国内地的肾脏移植情况进行动态、科学的分析，为国家监管部门制定移植相关的政策、法规提供了依据，为各移植中心提供了肾脏移植受者的科学管理工具。迄今为止，CSRKT 已成为中国器官移植领域最重要的信息化系统及肾脏移植学术交流平台之一。

一、肾脏移植医疗机构分布

截至 2020 年 12 月 31 日，中国共有 132 所医疗机构具备肾脏移植资质，医疗机构分布排名前十位的省（区、市）为广东（18 所）、北京（13 所）、山东（10 所）、湖南（9 所）、浙江（8 所）、上海（7 所）、广西（6 所）、河南（6 所）、湖北（6 所）和辽宁（5 所）（图 4-1）。

2015—2020 年，中国共实施肾脏移植 63 042 例，其中公民逝世后器官捐献（deceased donor，DD）肾脏移植 52 285 例，亲属间活体（living-related donor）肾脏移植 10 757 例。2020 年实施肾脏移植 11 037 例，总例数较 2019 年减少 9.0%；其中 DD 肾脏移植 9399 例，较 2019 年减少 9.5%；亲属间活体肾脏移植 1638 例，较 2019 年减少 5.6%（图 4-2）。

2020 年中国共实施肾脏相关的多器官联合移植 149 例，较 2019 年减少 33.5%（图 4-3），其中肝肾联合移植 39 例、胰肾联合移植 103 例、心肾联合移植 7 例。

2020 年实施肾脏相关的多器官联合移植例数排名前十位的省（区、市）为广东、山东、广西、天津、北京、上海、浙江、海南、河南、湖南和江苏（图 4-4），排名前十位的医疗机构依次为广州医科大学附属第二医院（59 例）、青岛大学附属医院（16 例）、广西医科大学第二附属医院（13 例）、中山大学附属第一医院（10 例）、天津市第一中心医院（8 例）、浙江大学医学院附属第一医院（4 例）、清华大学附属北京清华长庚医院（3 例）、复旦大学附属中山医院（3 例）、海南医学院第二附属医院（3 例）、河南中医药大学人民医院（郑州人民医院）（3 例）、中山大学附属第三医院（3 例）（表 4-1）。

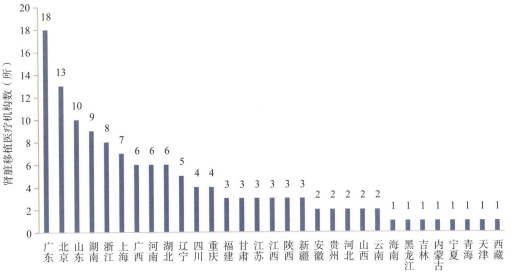

▲ 图 4-1 中国具有肾脏移植资质的医疗机构地理分布（截至 2020 年年底，不包含港澳台地区）

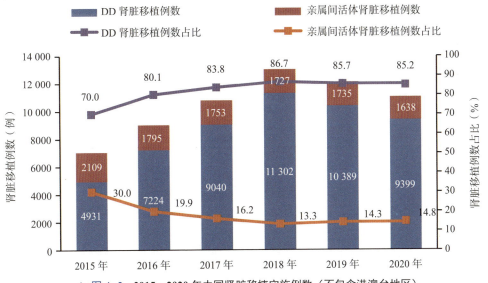

▲ 图 4-2 2015—2020 年中国肾脏移植实施例数（不包含港澳台地区）

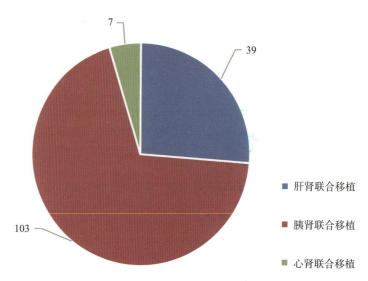

▲ 图 4-3　**2020 年中国肾脏相关的多器官联合移植实施例数（不包含港澳台地区）**

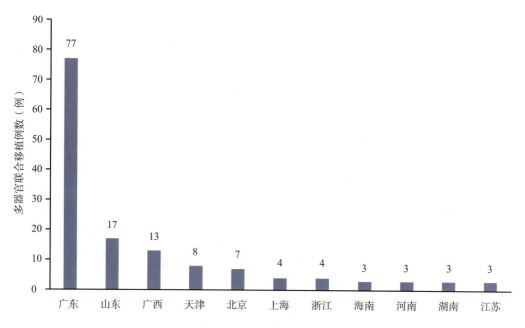

▲ 图 4-4　**2020 年中国肾脏相关的多器官联合移植实施例数前十位的省（区、市）（不包含港澳台地区）**

　　儿童（＜18 岁）肾脏移植近年得到关注，2020 年儿童肾脏移植例数占全国总例数的 2.7%（图 4-5）。

表 4-1 2020 年中国肾脏相关的多器官联合移植实施例数前十位的医疗机构（不包含港澳台地区）

地区	肾脏移植医院	例数
广东	广州医科大学附属第二医院	59
山东	青岛大学附属医院	16
广西	广西医科大学第二附属医院	13
广东	中山大学附属第一医院	10
天津	天津市第一中心医院	8
浙江	浙江大学医学院附属第一医院	4
北京	清华大学附属北京清华长庚医院	3
上海	复旦大学附属中山医院	3
海南	海南医学院第二附属医院	3
河南	河南中医药大学人民医院（郑州人民医院）	3
广东	中山大学附属第三医院	3

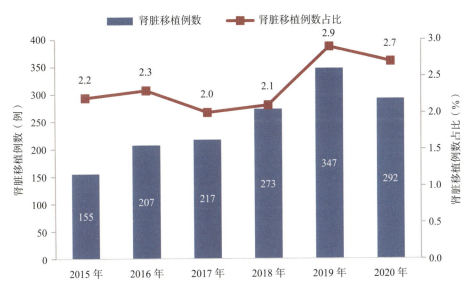

▲ 图 4-5 2015—2020 年中国儿童肾脏移植实施例数及占比（不包含港澳台地区）

2020 年实施肾脏移植例数排名前十位的省（区、市）依次为广东、浙江、山东、湖南、河南、上海、北京、湖北、四川和广西，各省（区、市）实施的肾脏移植例数分布见图 4-6。

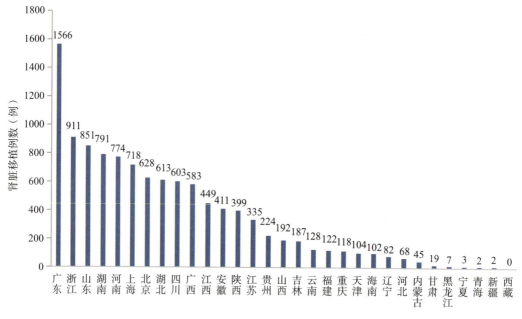

▲ 图 4-6　2020 年中国各省（区、市）肾脏移植例数分布（不包含港澳台地区）

2020 年实施肾脏移植 ≥ 250 例的医疗机构有 10 所，例数占比当年总例数的 32.6%；此外，200～249 例的有 5 所，100～199 例的有 25 所，50～99 例的有 22 所，10～49 例的有 34 所，1～9 例的有 18 所，有 18 所未开展肾脏移植（其中 7 所在 2018—2020 年连续 3 年未开展肾脏移植）。2020 年肾脏移植的各数量区间分布及例数占比见表 4-2。

例数区间	医疗机构数	例数占比（%）
表 4-2　2020 年中国肾脏移植数量区间分布及占比（不包含港澳台地区）		
≥ 250	10	32.6
200～249	5	9.9
100～199	25	31.6
50～99	22	15.4
10～49	34	9.7
1～9	18	0.8
0	18	0

　　2020 年中国肾脏移植手术的开展呈区域优势特征，有 9 个省（区、市）实施肾脏移植 ≥ 600 例，占全国当年总例数的 67.5%（表 4-3）。

表 4-3　2020 年中国各省（区、市）肾脏移植例数分布（不包含港澳台地区）		
例数区间	省（区、市）数	例数占比（%）
≥ 600	9	67.5
400～599	3	13.1
200～399	3	8.7
100～199	7	8.6
1～99	8	2.1
0	1	0

　　2020 年中国 DD 肾脏移植例数前十位的省（区、市）为广东、山东、湖南、浙江、上海、河南、北京、广西、湖北和江西，总计占比当年中国 DD 总例数的 75.3%（图 4-7）。排名前十位的医疗机构依次为上海交通大学医学院附属仁济医院

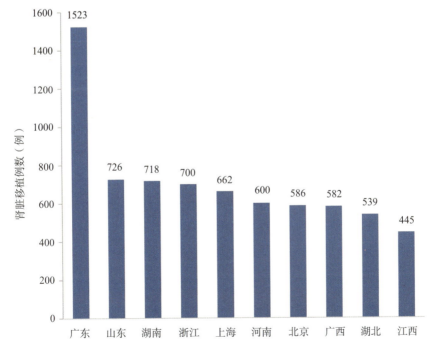

▲ 图 4-7　2020 年中国 DD 肾脏移植实施例数前十名的省（区、市）（不包含港澳台地区）

（412 例）、西安交通大学第一附属医院（365 例）、中山大学附属第一医院（344 例）、广州医科大学附属第二医院（290 例）、广西医科大学第二附属医院（288 例）、树兰（杭州）医院（279 例）、浙江大学医学院附属第一医院（257 例）、郑州大学第一附属医院（239 例）、青岛大学附属医院（223 例）、四川大学华西医院（222 例）（表 4-4）。

表 4-4　2020 年中国 DD 肾脏移植实施例数前十名医疗机构（不包含港澳台地区）

地　区	肾脏移植医院	例　数
上海	上海交通大学医学院附属仁济医院	412
陕西	西安交通大学第一附属医院	365
广东	中山大学附属第一医院	344
广东	广州医科大学附属第二医院	290
广西	广西医科大学第二附属医院	288
浙江	树兰（杭州）医院	279
浙江	浙江大学医学院附属第一医院	257
河南	郑州大学第一附属医院	239
山东	青岛大学附属医院	223
四川	四川大学华西医院	222

2020 年亲属间活体肾脏移植实施例数位居前十位的省（区、市）为四川、安徽、浙江、河南、山东、湖北、湖南、上海、广东和北京（图 4-8），位列前十位的医疗机构依次为四川大学华西医院（269 例）、中国科学技术大学附属第一医院（安徽省立医院）（233 例）、浙江大学医学院附属第一医院（201 例）、郑州大学第一附属医院（93 例）、安徽医科大学第一附属医院（64 例）、河南省人民医院（54 例）、中南大学湘雅第二医院（53 例）、华中科技大学同济医学院附属同济医院（49 例）、山东第一医科大学第一附属医院（山东省千佛山医院）（41 例）、四川省人民医院（40 例）（表 4-5）。

二、肾脏移植受者人口特征

对 2020 年中国内地实施的肾脏移植病例数据分析，结果显示，受者年龄为

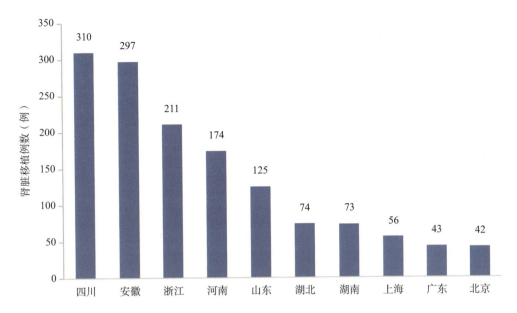

▲ 图 4-8　2020 年中国亲属间活体肾脏移植例数前十位的省（区、市）（不包含港澳台地区）

表 4-5　2020 年中国亲属间活体肾脏移植实施例数前十名医疗机构（不包含港澳台地区）		
地　区	肾脏移植医院	例　数
四川	四川大学华西医院	269
安徽	中国科学技术大学附属第一医院（安徽省立医院）	233
浙江	浙江大学医学院附属第一医院	201
河南	郑州大学第一附属医院	93
安徽	安徽医科大学第一附属医院	64
河南	河南省人民医院	54
湖南	中南大学湘雅二医院	53
湖北	华中科技大学同济医学院附属同济医院	49
山东	山东第一医科大学第一附属医院（山东省千佛山医院）	41
四川	四川省人民医院	40

（40.2±12.0）岁，BMI 为（22.0±3.4）kg/m^2，术前中位透析时间为 482 天，男性移植受者占比 69.3%，AB 血型移植受者占比最少（9.7%）（表 4-6）。

表 4-6　2020 年中国肾脏移植受者人口特征（不包含港澳台地区）	
变　量	均数 ± 标准差
受者年龄（岁）	40.2±12.0
BMI（kg/m^2）	22.0±3.4
透析时间	中位数（四分位间距）
术前透析时间（天）	482（244~1028）
受者血型	数量（占比，%）
O 型	3695（33.5）
A 型	3193（28.9）
B 型	3083（27.9）
AB 型	1066（9.7）
性　别	数量（占比，%）
男	7652（69.3）
女	3385（30.7）

受者年龄区间分布为儿童（＜18 岁）肾脏移植受者 292 例，占比 2.7%；18 岁及以上至 30 岁以下的受者 1792 例，占 16.2%；30 岁及以上至 50 岁以下的受者 6259 例，占 56.7%；50 岁及以上至 65 岁以下的受者 2520 例，占 22.8%；老年（≥65 岁）肾脏移植受者 174 例，占 1.6%。

三、肾脏移植质量安全分析

1. DD 肾脏移植供肾缺血时间

分别对 2020 年亲属间活体、DD 肾脏移植病例进行分析，供肾平均冷缺血时间不超过 6h（表 4-7）。99.9% 的亲属间活体肾脏移植和 99.7% 的 DD 肾脏移植其供肾冷缺血时间≤24h；98.4% 的亲属间活体肾脏移植和 83.8% 的 DD 肾脏移植其供肾热缺血时间≤10min（表 4-8）。

表 4-7　2020 年亲属间活体、DD 肾脏移植供肾缺血时间（不包含港澳台地区）

变　量	亲属间活体（均值 ± 标准差）	DD（均值 ± 标准差）
供肾冷缺血时间（h）	1.9±1.2	5.8±3.9
供肾热缺血时间（min）	3.1±2.3	6.4±5.1

表 4-8　2020 年亲属间活体、DD 肾脏移植供肾缺血时间占比（不包含港澳台地区）

变　量	亲属间活体（%）	DD（%）
供肾冷缺血时间≤24h	99.9	99.7
供肾热缺血时间≤10min	98.4	83.8

2. 肾脏移植前后受者血清肌酐值的变化情况

2020 年全国共实施 11 037 例肾脏移植手术，根据 CSRKT 要求，分析 4 个随访时间点（术前、术后 30 天、180 天、360 天）的亲属间活体肾脏移植、DD 肾脏移植受者的血清肌酐平均值（表 4-9）。

表 4-9　2020 年亲属间活体、DD 肾脏移植受者术前、术后的血清肌酐平均值（不包含港澳台地区）

时间点	亲属间活体（μmol/L）	DD（μmol/L）
术前	1012.0	932.5
术后 30 天	119.2	145.7
术后 180 天	116.2	122.9
术后 360 天	117.3	115.7

3. 肾脏移植术后不良事件概况

肾脏移植术后不良事件主要包括移植肾功能延迟恢复、急性排斥反应、感染、移植受者死亡、移植肾丢失等。对 2020 年病例的随访资料进行分析，主要不良事件发生率（表 4-10 和表 4-11）。受者术后 30 天内死亡率为 0.3%，未见亲属间活体捐献者术后 30 天内重大并发症发生者。

表 4-10　2020 年中国肾脏移植术后不良事件发生率（不包含港澳台地区）

不良事件	亲属间活体（%）	DD（%）
移植肾功能延迟恢复	2.4	12.2
急性排斥反应	1.8	4.8
感染	1.1	2.5
移植受者死亡	0.7	1.7
移植肾全因丢失	1.0	3.6

表 4-11　2020 年中国胰肾联合移植术后不良事件发生率（不包含港澳台地区）

不良事件	总体发生率（%）
移植肾功能延迟恢复	8.7
急性排斥反应	9.7
感染	6.8
移植受者死亡	12.6
移植肾全因丢失	12.6

4. 肾脏移植受者、移植物生存分析

选取 2015—2020 年期间全国范围内开展的肾脏移植共计 63 042 例，进行移植受者 / 移植物（以下简称"人 / 肾"）的生存分析，结果如下。

(1) 移植术后 1 年生存率：亲属间活体肾脏移植的 1 年人 / 肾生存率为 99.3% / 98.7%；DD 肾脏移植的 1 年人 / 肾生存率为 97.8%/95.8%（表 4-12）。

(2) 移植术后 3 年生存率：亲属间活体肾脏移植的 3 年人 / 肾生存率为 98.8%/96.8%；DD 肾脏移植的 3 年人 / 肾生存率为 96.8%/93.2%（表 4-12）。

表 4-12　中国肾脏移植术后生存率（不包含港澳台地区）

供体类别	术后 1 年		术后 3 年	
	移植受者（%）	移植物（%）	移植受者（%）	移植物（%）
亲属间活体肾脏	99.3	98.7	98.8	96.8
DD 肾脏	97.8	95.8	96.8	93.2

四、特点与展望

1. DD 肾脏移植是当今主要的移植类型

我国肾脏移植事业已进入了一个全新的良性发展阶段。在过去的 5 年中，DD 肾脏移植例数占比均在 80% 以上，2020 年则为 85.2%，以广东、山东、湖南、浙江和上海等省市位居前列，区域优势明显。儿童肾脏移植以广东、河南和上海等省市开展较多。儿童肾脏捐献继续得到应用与关注。

器官的区域分配原则及器官转运绿色通道的建立，缩短了 DD 肾脏移植的供肾冷缺血时间。亲属间活体肾脏移植和 DD 肾脏移植的 1 年、3 年移植肾生存率满意。2020 年肾脏相关的多器官联合移植 149 例，其中 69.1% 为胰肾联合移植，在广东、山东、广西、天津和北京开展较多。

2. 持续开展肾脏移植质量控制与质量提升工程

质控中心的宗旨是以建设符合中国肾脏移植学科发展特点的 CSRKT 为基石，发挥行业引领作用，加强人体器官移植医疗质量的管理，实现全国肾脏移植医疗质量和服务水平的持续改进，缩小各移植中心的医疗差距，一系列质控标准与技术规范由此出台，并在过去两年内持续更新，内容涉及肾脏移植的各技术领域，具有极大的临床指导意义，从而实现从医学质量评价（控制）到医疗质量提升的良性循环，不断推进我国肾脏移植事业的发展。

3. 关注肾脏移植研究热点并取得突破性进展

在未来很长时间内，器官移植供体短缺和移植排斥反应依然是制约肾脏移植发展的关键因素。多年来，国内学者致力于将免疫学、干细胞和基因工程等领域的成果与器官移植紧密联系起来，大力开展基础与临床研究，为进一步优化肾脏移植医疗质量提供了理论和实践依据。在缺血再灌注损伤、急性排斥反应、慢性移植物失功、肾脏纤维化、边缘供肾的维护与利用、移植相关病毒感染、肾脏移植后临床指标监测及预警、低体重婴幼儿双供肾成人肾脏移植等方面，已取得突破性进展。

第 5 章 中国心脏移植

本章内容主要基于中国心脏移植注册系统（China Heart Transplant Registry, CHTR）数据分析，统计范围是中国内地，不包含港澳台地区。

CHTR 是由国家卫生健康委员会建立的国家心脏移植注册系统，要求全国具有心脏移植资质的医疗机构必须及时、完整地向其填报移植相关信息。CHTR 主要数据内容包括受体基本情况、心脏供体情况、移植术中情况、免疫抑制剂应用情况、移植近期和远期结果。CHTR 通过对中国内地的心脏移植情况进行动态、科学地分析，定期发布各心脏移植中心手术量、数据质量和临床质量，并基于移植数据，发布心脏供体获取和保存、组织配型和移植围术期管理等方面的结果和经验，为国家监管部门制定移植相关的政策、法规提供科学依据。

一、心脏移植医疗机构分布

截至 2020 年 12 月 31 日，中国共有 56 所医疗机构具备心脏移植资质，心脏移植医院数量排名前十位的省（区、市）依次为广东（6 所）、浙江（6 所）、北京（5 所）、湖北（5 所）、河南（3 所）、天津（3 所）、云南（3 所）、福建（2 所）、广西（2 所）、辽宁（2 所）、山东（2 所）、上海（2 所）和四川（2 所）。而西藏、甘肃、贵州、江西和吉林等地区尚无心脏移植医院（图 5-1）。

CHTR 数据显示，2015—2020 年全国上报心脏移植手术共 2819 例（图 5-2）。2020 年共有 38 家心脏移植医疗机构实施并上报心脏移植手术 557 例，移植例数比 2019 年减少了 18.0%，其中儿童（＜ 18 岁）心脏移植 52 例，心肺联合移植 7 例。各省（区、市）心脏移植例数分布如图 5-3 所示。2020 年，除港澳台地区外，中国心脏移植例数排名前十位的医疗机构依次为中国医学科学院阜外医院（78 例）、华中科技大学同济医学院附属协和医院（73 例）、广东省人民医院（54 例）、郑州市第七人民医院（44 例）、复旦大学附属中山医院（43 例）、浙江大学医学院附属第一医院（26 例）、福建医科大学附属协和医院（25 例）、南京市第一医院（22 例）、中山大学孙逸仙纪念医院（18 例）和武汉亚洲心脏病医院（16 例）（图5-4）。

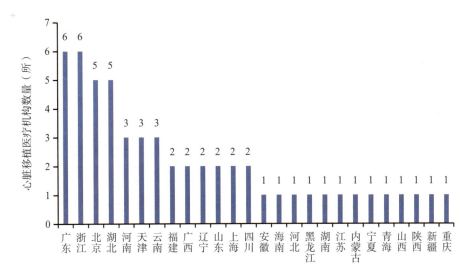

▲ 图 5-1　2020 年中国具有心脏移植医疗机构分布情况（不包含港澳台地区）

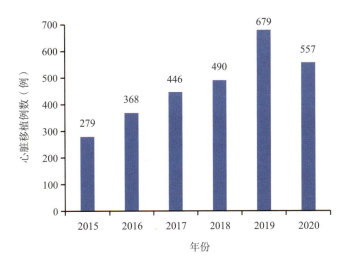

▲ 图 5-2　2015—2020 年中国心脏移植例数（不包含港澳台地区）

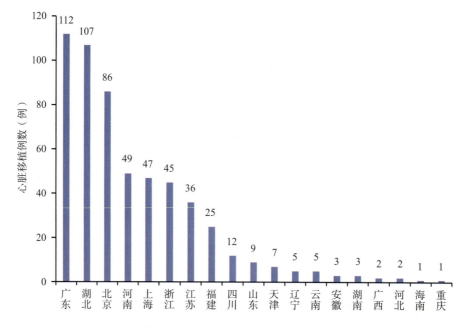

▲ 图 5-3　**2020 年中国各省（区、市）心脏移植例数分布（不包含港澳台地区）**

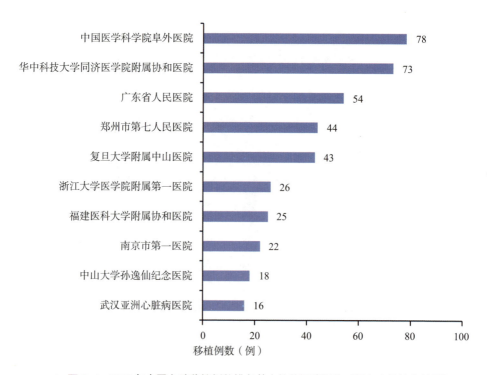

▲ 图 5-4　**2020 年中国心脏移植例数排名前十位的医疗机构（不包含港澳台地区）**

二、心脏移植受者人口特征

2020 年，心脏移植受者年龄中位数为 50.0 岁，其中，男性受者比例为 74.7%；受者 BMI 中位数为 22.2（kg/m²）。移植受者血型中 O 型占 30.8%，A 型占 30.5%，B 型占 28.3%，AB 型占 10.4%。成人移植受者年龄中位数为 52.0 岁，男性占比 76.1%；儿童移植受者年龄中位数为 10.5 岁，男性占比 56.6%（表 5-1）。心脏移植受者病因以非缺血性心肌病和冠心病为主，占比分别为 74.4% 和 15.5%，其次为心脏瓣膜病（4.4%）和先天性心脏病（3.0%）。成人受者病因以非缺血性心肌病（73.3%）和冠心病为主（16.9%）；儿童受者病因以非缺血性心肌病（84.9%）和先天性心脏病（11.3%）为主。

表 5-1 2020 年中国心脏移植受者人口特征（不包含港澳台地区）			
变量	总体移植受者（N=557）	成人移植受者（N=505）	儿童移植受者（N=52）
年龄中位数，IQR（岁）	50.0（34.0～59.0）	52.0（40.0～59.0）	10.5（3.5～12.5）
男性占比（%）	74.7	76.1	56.6
体重中位数，IQR（kg）	62.3（54.0～70.0）	54.3（56.0～71.7）	26.0（16.0～40.0）
身高中位数，IQR（cm）	169.0（161.0～172.0）	170.0（163.0～173.0）	140.0（110.0～160.0）
BMI 中位数，IQR（kg/m²）	22.2（19.6～24.6）	22.5（20.4～24.8）	14.9（13.0～18.0）
心脏移植病因占比（%）			
非缺血性心肌病	74.4	73.3	84.9
冠心病	15.5	16.9	1.9
先天性心脏病	3.0	2.0	11.3
心脏瓣膜病	4.4	4.9	0
其他疾病	2.7	2.9	1.9

IQR. 四分位间距

三、心脏移植质量安全分析

1. 心脏缺血时间

2020 年，全国心脏移植的缺血时间分布如图 5-5 所示。2020 年我国心脏移植心脏缺血时间中位数为 3.7h，与 2019 年缺血时间中位数 4.0h 相比有所下降。心脏移植缺血时间≤ 6h 的移植受者占比为 83.4%，略低于 2019 年的 84.4%。

2. 术中术后机械辅助的应用率

2020 年，全国心脏移植术中术后机械辅助的使用情况见图 5-6。其中，2020 年主动脉球囊反搏（intra-aortic balloon pump，IABP）的应用率为 19.0%，体外膜肺氧合（extracorporeal membrane oxygenation，ECMO）的应用率为 12.7%，连续性肾脏替代治疗（continuous renal replacement therapy，CRRT）的应用率为 21.2%，分别高于 2019 年的 18.0%、10.0% 和 16.4%（图 5-6）。

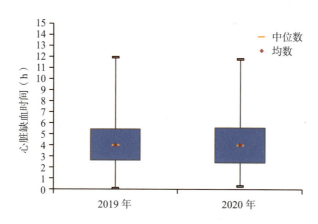

▲ 图 5-5　2019 年和 2020 年中国心脏移植心脏缺血时间情况（不包含港澳台地区）

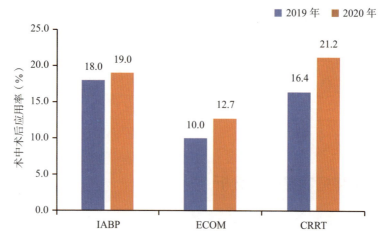

▲ 图 5-6　2019 年和 2020 年中国心脏移植术中术后机械辅助应用情况（不包含港澳台地区）

3. 术后机械通气时间

2020 年我国心脏移植术后机械通气时间中位数为 36h（图 5-7），大于 2019 年术后机械通气时间中位数（27h）。2019 年术后机械通气时间≤ 48h 的移植受者占比为 71.5%，2020 年的占比为 63.7%。

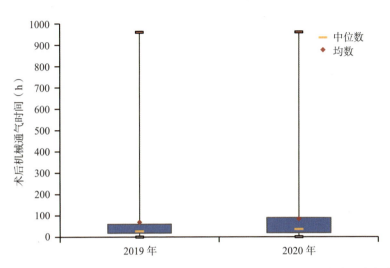

▲ 图 5-7　**2019 年和 2020 年中国心脏移植术后机械通气时间情况（不包含港澳台地区）**

4. 术后院内生存情况

2020 年，我国心脏移植受者院内存活率为 88.5%。心脏移植受者术后感染发生率为 26.6%，其他术后主要并发症分别为心搏骤停（5.7%）、二次开胸（5.7%）、气管切开（6.3%）和二次插管（7.9%）。在心脏移植受者院内死亡原因情况中，多器官衰竭和移植心脏衰竭共占早期死亡原因的 60% 以上（表 5-2）。

<table>
<tr><th colspan="4">表 5-2　2020 年心脏移植受者术后院内生存情况</th></tr>
<tr><th rowspan="3">变　量</th><th colspan="3">率 / 构成比（%）</th></tr>
<tr><th>总体移植受者
（N=557）</th><th>成人移植受者
（N=505）</th><th>儿童移植受者
（N=52）</th></tr>
<tr><td>院内存活</td><td>88.5</td><td>88.0</td><td>92.3</td></tr>
<tr><td>术后并发症</td><td></td><td></td><td></td></tr>
<tr><td>术后感染</td><td>23.4</td><td>22.9</td><td>28.3</td></tr>
<tr><td>心搏骤停</td><td>5.7</td><td>5.5</td><td>7.6</td></tr>
</table>

（续表）

变 量	率 / 构成比（%）		
	总体移植受者 （N=557）	成人移植受者 （N=505）	儿童移植受者 （N=52）
二次开胸	5.7	5.9	3.8
气管切开	6.3	6.7	1.9
二次插管	7.9	8.4	3.8
院内死亡原因			
多器官衰竭	34.4	34.5	33
移植心脏衰竭	15.6	27.6	50
感染	26.6	12.1	17
其他	23.5	25.8	0

5. 生存分析

2015—2020 年全国心脏移植术后 30 天、术后 1 年和术后 3 年的生存率分别为 92.6%、85.3% 和 80.4%。其中，成人心脏移植术后的 30 天生存率、1 年生存率和 3 年生存率分别为 92.5%、85.3% 和 80.4%；儿童心脏移植术后的 30 天生存率、1 年生存率和 3 年生存率分别为 94.5%、91.0% 和 84.0%（表 5–3）。

表 5–3　2015—2020 年心脏移植术后生存率			
	术后 30 天生存率（%）	术后 1 年生存率（%）	术后 3 年生存率（%）
总体移植受者	92.6	85.3	80.4
成人移植受者	92.5	85.3	80.4
儿童移植受者	94.5	91.0	84.0

四、特点与展望

受新冠肺炎疫情影响，2020 年全国心脏移植例数比 2019 年下降了 18%，但仍比 2018 年增加了 14%。中国医学科学院阜外医院、华中科技大学同济医学院附属协和医院、广东省人民医院三家心脏移植中心 2020 年移植例数大于 50 例，郑州市第七人民医院、复旦大学附属中山医院全年移植例数也超过 40 例，以上移植中心在全国抗击疫情的背景下保持了较高的医疗服务能力，为我国心脏移植等待者们提供了较为稳定的医疗可及性。然而，排名前十位的心脏移植中心都集中在我国的中东部地区，心脏移植地区间发展差异仍需进一步缩小。

在心脏供体缺血时间方面，得益于中国人体器官分配与共享计算机系统的高效运行及各家移植医疗团队的不懈努力，2020 年心脏缺血时间 ≤ 6h 的例数占比与 2019 年的数据接近，但与欧美国家相比仍有较大差距，需要进一步优化心脏供体分配制度，加强供体获取效率和转运合作。心脏移植患者术后机械通气时间中位数和 < 48h 的比例均差于 2019 年，这提示在供体选择维护和受者围术期管理方面需要进一步提高医疗质量。

心脏移植术后结局方面，2020 年我国心脏移植院内死亡率高于 2019 年，提示在供受者评估及围术期管理等方面进行质量控制和提升，进一步降低院内死亡率。

展望未来，中国心脏移植质控中心将进一步完善中国心脏移植注册系统，鼓励和帮扶新获取心脏移植资质的医院，并通过开展一系列心脏移植医疗质量改善项目，持续改善我国心脏移植医疗质量。

第6章 中国肺脏移植

本章内容主要基于中国肺脏移植注册系统（China Lung Transplantation Registry，CLuTR）中的数据分析，统计范围是中国内地，不包含港澳台地区。

CLuTR 是由国家卫生健康委员会建立的国家肺脏移植注册系统，全面及时地收集了受者术前、捐献者、受者手术、术后及随访信息。通过对中国内地的肺脏移植情况进行动态、科学地分析，为国家监管部门制定移植相关政策、法规提供依据。

一、肺脏移植医疗机构分布

截至 2020 年 12 月 31 日，除港澳台地区外，全国共有 43 所医疗机构取得肺脏移植资质，覆盖全国 21 个省（区、市），其中医疗机构前十位的省（区、市）依次为北京（5 所）、广东（5 所）、湖北（4 所）、浙江（4 所）、天津（3 所）、上海（3 所）、辽宁（2 所）、四川（2 所）、河南（2 所）和广西（2 所）。河北、山西、吉林、江西、重庆、贵州、西藏、甘肃、青海和宁夏地区尚无医疗机构取得肺脏移植资质（图 6-1）。

2015 年 1 月 1 日至 2020 年 12 月 31 日，CLuTR 共上报肺脏移植手术 2026 例，各年度开展肺脏移植手术分别为 118 例、204 例、299 例、403 例、489 例和 513 例（图 6-2），呈逐年上升趋势。

2020 年，有 29 个中心开展了肺脏移植手术。手术数量居前十位的中心依次为无锡市人民医院（156 例）、中日友好医院（77 例）、广州医科大学附属第一医院（76 例）、上海市肺科医院（40 例）、郑州大学第一附属医院（39 例）、浙江大学医学院附属第二医院（26 例）、浙江大学医学院附属第一医院（18 例）、河南省人民医院（15 例）、四川省人民医院（12 例）和中国科学技术大学附属第一医院（安徽省立医院）（9 例）（图 6-3）。

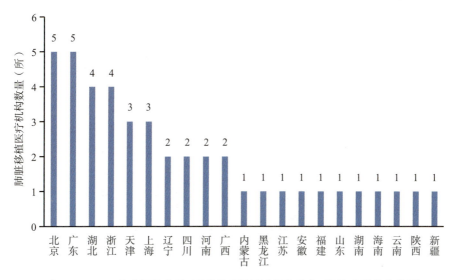

▲ 图 6-1　2020 年中国具有肺脏移植资质的医疗机构分布（不包含港澳台地区）

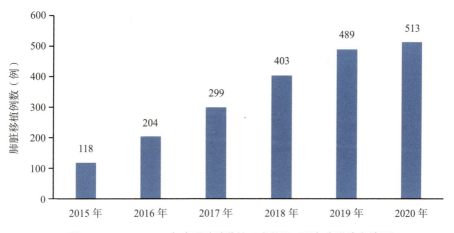

▲ 图 6-2　2015—2020 年中国肺脏移植手术数量（不包含港澳台地区）

二、肺脏移植受者人口特征

2020 年我国肺脏移植单、双肺冷缺血时间中位数（IQR）分别为 6.5h（5.0～7.5h）和 8.5h（7.0～9.5h）。单肺冷缺血时间＜ 2h、2～4h、4～6h、6～8h 及 ≥ 8h 的比例分比为 4.8%、16.3%、22.3%、48.2% 和 8.4%；双肺冷缺血时间相应比例分别为 0.0%、3.7%、15.4%、23.4% 和 57.5%（图 6-4）。

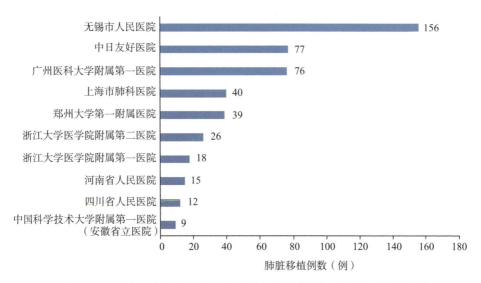

▲ 图 6-3　**2020 年度中国肺脏移植例数前十位的医疗机构（不包含港澳台地区）**

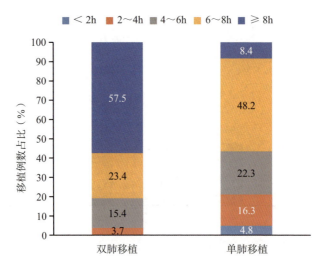

▲ 图 6-4　**2020 年单、双肺冷缺血时间（不包含港澳台地区）**

2020 年我国肺脏移植受者男性占 66.8%；年龄为（54.9±12.8）岁，60 岁以上占 48.0%。BMI 为（20.7±3.5）kg/m²；O、A、B 及 AB 血型分别占比 31.3%、29.2%、28.7% 及 9.7%。移植前 32.2% 的受者使用过激素药物，13.8% 的受者在 ICU 住院；心功能状态方面，日常活动完全受限（NYHA Ⅳ）及病情严重需住院治疗的比例分别为 24.3% 和 16.1%（表 6-1）。

表 6-1　2020 年肺脏移植受者人口特征（不包含港澳台地区）			
变　量	占比（%）	变　量	占比（%）
性别		血型	
男	66.8	O 型	31.3
女	33.2	A 型	29.2
年龄（岁）		B 型	28.7
＜ 18	1.1	AB 型	9.7
18—35	8.5	激素药物治疗史	
36—49	16.1	有	32.2
50—59	26.3	无	67.8
60—64	27.3	移植前住院情况	
≥ 65	20.7	ICU	13.8
BMI 分级（kg/m^2）		普通住院	70.1
＜ 18.5	27.9	未住院	14.7
18.6～23.9	51.5	移植前心功能状态	
≥ 24.0	17.1	无活动限制（NYHA Ⅰ/Ⅱ）	1.8
		日常活动部分受限（NYHA Ⅲ）	53.4
		日常活动完全受限（NYHA Ⅳ）	24.3
		病情严重需住院治疗	16.1

2020 年我国肺脏移植受者原发病中以特发性肺间质纤维化、慢性阻塞性肺疾病、继发性肺间质纤维化和尘肺为主，分别占 38.2%、21.8%、13.1% 和 10.1%。此外，支气管扩张症、肺动脉高压、闭塞性细支气管炎、淋巴管平滑肌瘤病和移植肺功能衰竭分别占 5.7%、3.1%、1.5%、1.4% 和 1.1%（图 6-5）。

三、肺脏移植质量安全分析

1. 手术方式

2020 年我国肺脏移植术中单、双肺移植分别占 37.2% 和 62.8%。急诊肺移植占

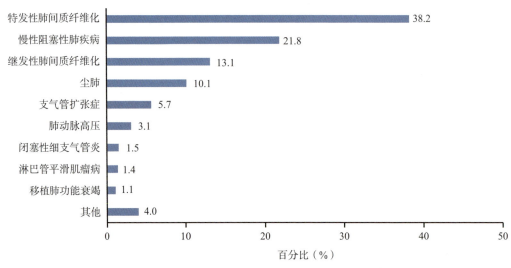

▲ 图 6-5　2020 年我国肺脏移植受者原发病分布（不包含港澳台地区）

15.0%，术中使用体外膜肺氧合（extracorporeal membrane oxygenation，ECMO）的比例为 68.7%。

2. 术中输血

术中输血量的中位数（IQR）为 1012.5ml（520.0～1840.0ml），＜ 500ml、500～999ml、1000～1499ml、1500～1999ml 和 ≥ 2000ml 的比例分别为 24.2%、20.3%、20.3%、11.6% 和 23.6%。

3. 术后早期（＜ 30 天）并发症

术后早期并发症主要包括感染（64.6%）、肾功能不全（29.4%）、原发性肺移植物失功（13.2%）、气管吻合口病变（10.3%）和急性排斥反应（5.9%）（图 6-6）。

4. 出院时状态

2020 年我国肺脏移植受者住院时间中位数（IQR）为 31.0 天（17.0～51.0 天），围术期存活率为 83.5%。受者围术期死因主要为肺部感染导致的休克或呼吸循环衰竭（41.3%）、多器官功能衰竭（30.7%）、心源性猝死（8.0%）和失血性休克（5.3%）（图 6-7）。

5. 术后生存状况

我国双肺移植受者术后围术期（＜ 30 天）、3 个月、6 个月、1 年及 3 年生存率分别为 80.5%、69.9%、66.6%、62.7% 和 54.1%，单肺移植受者相应生存率分别为 83.9%、76.8%、72.1%、65.8% 和 54.0%，单肺移植受者近期生存率优于双肺移植受者（表 6-2）。

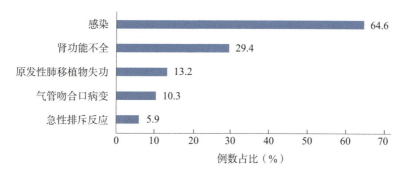

▲ 图 6-6　**2020 年我国肺脏移植受者围术期并发症（不包含港澳台地区）**

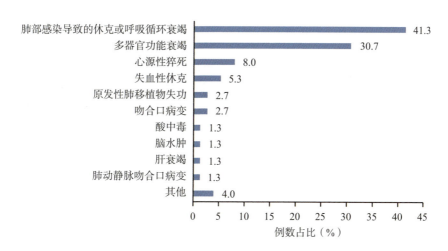

▲ 图 6-7　**2020 年我国肺脏移植受者围手术期死因（不包含港澳台地区）**

表 6-2　中国肺脏移植术后受者生存率（不包含港澳台地区）					
	围术期（< 30 天）	3 个月	6 个月	1 年	3 年
双肺（%）	80.5	69.9	66.6	62.7	54.1
单肺（%）	83.9	76.8	72.1	65.8	54.0

四、特点与展望

近年来，国家肺脏移植质控中心不断完善肺移植临床诊疗体系，推广规范化肺移植技术。2020 年我国肺移植例数相比 2019 年继续保持了全国肺移植数量上升势头。2020 年，在重症新冠肺炎患者肺移植领域取得了较大突破，但急诊肺移植、术后感染、原发性移植物失功、心源性猝死、肾功能不全等术后并发症发生率仍然较高。

2020年新冠肺炎疫情期间，我国开创性探索开展了全球首例新型冠状病毒肺炎终末期呼吸衰竭患者双肺移植手术，并制订了"高选择性、高防护性"新冠肺炎肺移植手术原则，为此类新冠肺炎终末期呼吸衰竭患者的救治提供了中国经验。

急诊肺移植患者病情危重、时间仓促，移植存在更大风险，术后发生排斥反应及原发性移植物失功的危险较高，术后围术期生存率及近远期生存率也更低。因此，应进一步推动肺移植术前评估制度，严格把关受者的移植禁忌证和适应证。

对感染控制，应继续推进全程化、多环节的感控机制建设，从术前评估、供者质量维护、手术操作和术后管理多个层面做好感染预防和控制工作。对原发性移植物失功的防治，应充分把好供体质量关，对身体功能较差的受者可考虑使用体外循环辅助技术或适当延长 ECMO 转流时间。对心源性猝死的防治，要重视术前受者心功能状态的评估，术后要动态监测心功能状态，对心功能异常者，要予以积极处理。对肾功能不全的防治，要重视药物浓度和肾功能指标的监测，尤其要注意药物之间的相互作用，尽量避免加重肾脏负担。

与国际肺移植情况相比，我国肺移植受者年龄大、病情危重、手术难度大、肺纤维化患者多，且公民逝世后捐献供肺的呼吸机使用时间长、冷缺血时间长，导致了我国肺移植患者生存率低于国际心肺移植协会报道数据。下一步工作将根据修订的肺脏移植技术临床应用质量控制指标加大对各移植中心质量的监测，继续完善肺移植流程和技术规范，打造多学科联合的肺移植团队，持续提升肺移植质量。

第7章 中国器官移植技术进展与创新

一、无缺血器官移植技术

现有的"冷移植"技术体系下，器官在血管离断至重新吻合全过程的血供完全中断，缺血损伤及恢复血流后的再灌注损伤不可避免，可引起原发性移植物无功能、早期移植物功能不全等严重并发症，成为影响移植疗效和器官利用率的主要原因。何晓顺教授团队经过8年的探索，研制出了全球首台体外多器官修复系统（Life-X），可为离体器官创造接近生理状态的灌注压、温度、氧合及营养支持，首次实现了多器官在"离体状态"下长时间保持功能与活力，并可修复受损器官功能，取代了传统冷保存技术。基于多器官修复系统的技术创新，何晓顺教授团队进一步全面革新移植手术方式，保证了器官血管离断、再吻合过程中，器官血流不中断，于2017年成功实施了全球首例"无缺血肝脏移植"术。复流后移植肝未出现细胞凋亡、炎症因子释放和损伤通路激活等缺血损伤现象，术后天冬氨酸氨基转移酶（aspartate aminotransferase，AST）峰值较传统技术下降74.7%，丙氨酸氨基转移酶（alanine aminotransferase，ALT）下降77.7%，原发性移植物无功能（primary graft non-function，PNF）从3.1%降至0%，早期移植物功能不全（EAD）从50.0%降至5.3%，复流后综合征从81.8%降至6.5%，ICU停留时间从43.5h缩短至34h，1年受体生存率较常规技术提高了9.8%。由于整个移植过程中器官保持正常的血供与温度，避免了传统"冷移植"中低温对心、肺、肾等重要脏器功能的影响，大大降低了手术风险。2018年成功实施了全球首例"无缺血肾脏移植"术。

二、我国自体肝移植情况介绍

1989年德国Pichlmayr教授首次报道自体肝移植（auto liver transplantation，

ALT）技术，国内黄洁夫教授于 2005 年首次采用 ALT 治疗肝棘球蚴病，开创国内 ALT 的先河。迄今国外报道的病例总数尚未突破 200 例。我国专家学者在董家鸿教授、郑树森教授、叶啟发教授、温浩教授及四川华西医院等团队的技术引领下，陆续开展 ALT 手术已 300 余例，为国际范围内的最大病例组。自体肝移植是对采用常规外科手术不能切除的肝内占位性病变，应用肝移植技术，在肝脏灌注和转流的条件下，离体或半离体切除肝脏病灶，修整保留肝脏，再将保留肝脏植入原位，达到根治肝占位性病变的外科技术。该技术为常规不能手术切除的肝脏良恶性占位性病灶或严重肝脏外伤提供了手术治愈的可能。相对于同种异体肝移植，该技术无须异体肝脏，不需要服用免疫抑制剂，减少了药费和相关并发症，具有重要的社会和经济效益。叶啟发教授团队在自体肝移植的术前肝功能评估、肝脏切除比率的计算、术中灌注技术与保存方法以及保留肝功能维护等方面制订了技术规范，达成自体肝移植国际共识，发挥了推广自体肝移植技术的关键作用。

三、器官移植的免疫抑制剂精准治疗

钙调磷酸酶抑制剂（CNIs）他克莫司的应用大大降低了移植术后排斥反应的发生，提高了移植器官生存率。但 CNIs 治疗窗窄、个体间药动力学参数差异显著，不同个体适宜的给药剂量呈现显著差别，迫切需要"量体裁衣"的精准诊治方案。研究表明，药物代谢酶 CYP3A5 的基因多态性是造成患者血浆中他克莫司浓度差异的主要原因。*CYP3A5* 基因第 3 内含子内 22893 位存在 6986A > G 突变（RS776746，CYP3A5*3），该 SNP 可导致 CYP3A5 mRNA 异常剪接，引起终止密码子过早剪切 CYP3A5 蛋白，从而使其失去酶活性。CYP3A5*3 纯合子个体肝脏和肠道 CYP3A5 蛋白表达和活性显著下降。活性降低导致他克莫司血药浓度升高。临床药物基因组学实施联盟指南建议携带 CYP3A5*3 基因型的移植患者减少他克莫司的用药剂量，以避免发生药物不良反应。

自 2008 年始，国家卫生健康委员会移植医学工程技术中心叶啟发教授联合中国工程院周宏灏院士，带领武汉大学中南医院与中南大学湘雅三医院移植团队，采用 Sanger 测序法检测移植前患者 *CYP3A5* 基因型，根据不同基因型推荐他克莫司初始给药剂量。目前已经完成 2120 余例，发现 CYP3A5*3 纯合子个体的突变频率高达 52.90%，提示检测群体中高达 50% 以上的患者，他克莫司剂量需要减量 50%。根据基因型给对应初始剂量后，患者 7 天内他克莫司用药浓度达标率从 37.5% 提高至 77.8%，他克莫司剂量需要调整的比例从 55.6% 降至 22.3%。3 个月内排斥反应发生率和药物中毒不良反应发生率表现明显下降。移植术后 7 天内，推荐初始给药剂量组中，快代谢型组他克莫司药费显著低于对照组。慢代谢型组他克莫司药物显著高于对照组。但是两组的排斥反应治疗费用均显著降低。

目前，此技术已在全国范围内移植中心推广应用，且已经研发出精准、快速、高效、便捷、经济的检测 CYP3A5*3 基因多态性的试剂盒，将为实现 CNIs 药物临床个体化治疗，提高移植预后起到积极的推动作用。

四、腔静脉右心房吻合肝移植新技术

腔静脉 – 心房吻合肝移植（vana cava and atrium anastomotic liver transplantation，VC-AALT）系叶啟发教授团队于 1996 年开创，用于治疗布 – 加综合征（Budd-Chiari syndrome，BCS），可防止 BCS 复发，取得了良好的疗效。

该技术的核心是根据下腔静脉不同病变，保留受者肝后下腔静脉，或切除肝后下腔静脉，或仅于心房下结扎肝上腔静脉，或在 ECMO 转流下（肿瘤蔓延心房）完成连同肝后腔静脉与病肝的切除，然后完成供肝肝上腔静脉与右心房端 – 侧吻合，供肝肝下腔静脉与受体腔静脉吻合。

单中心已实施 30 余例，长期随访表明 1 年、3 年、5 年生存率分别为 88.89%、83.33%、77.78%。国外仅见于 2018 年报道 4 例，中国早于国外 22 年。作者根据 BCS 病理进展不同先后创建了桥式背驮式肝移植（bridge-piggyback liver transplantation，B-PBLT）、心房悬吊式肝移植（atrial suspension liver transplantation，ASLT）、腔静脉切除桥式肝移植（vena cava resection bridge liver transplantation，VCRBLT）、ECMO 转流 VC-AALT 和辅助性原旁位心房悬吊式肝移植。

腔静脉 – 心房吻合系列技术应用于 BCS，防止了 BCS 复发（经典式肝移植、背驮式肝移植均因肝后、肝上腔静脉、肝静脉病变不能切除而复发），终末期肝硬化、肝肿瘤合并肝后腔静脉海绵变、腔静脉闭塞、腔静脉血栓、肿瘤蔓延右心房等疾病开拓了新技术路径。也为儿童代谢性疾病、原旁位辅助肝移植、静脉回流重建困难的患者开辟了新技术。

五、劈离式肝移植

1.劈离式肝移植简介

边缘性供肝、活体部分供肝、心脏死亡器官捐献（donation after cardiac death，DCD）供肝等增加了供肝来源，但供肝短缺问题仍未得到解决，制约了我国肝脏移植事业的发展。1984年，Bismuth等报道了首例将成人减体积肝移植左叶供肝用于儿童受体的报道，减体积肝移植逐渐成为儿童肝移植的金标准。以此为基础，一肝两用的思路逐渐清晰。1988年，Pichlmayr等开展了世界首例劈离式肝移植（split liver transplantation，SLT），将1例完整供肝劈离为两个具有独立解剖和功能的移植物后，分别移植给1例儿童受体和1例成年人受体。同年，Bismuth等首次使用SLT将1例供肝移植给了2例成人受体。与活体肝移植（living donor liver transplantation，LDLT）相比，SLT供肝来源于公民逝世后器官捐献，对于肝移植外科技术的要求更高，但不会对供体造成外科手术风险，且一肝两用能够更合理地分配供体肝脏。在开展SLT的初期，国际上各移植中心患者术后预后并不理想，生存率及并发症发生率也不尽相同。此外，SLT术后胆道并发症较全肝移植显著增高，早期可达40%。但是，随着供受体匹配与脉管分配原则在各中心逐渐形成共识，肝脏劈离和移植技术的成熟，国际上各中心SLT受者存活率逐渐上升，1年生存率达到80%～90%，血管及胆管并发症也显著下降。

2.我国劈离式肝移植的发展与现状

自2015年开始，我国全面进入公民逝世后器官捐献来源供体时代，供肝短缺问题依然严重，客观上推动了各中心对于SLT技术的开展。据统计，2015年、2016年中国大陆SLT开展数量分别为34例和41例，此后各中心供肝劈离例数逐年递增，2018年达140例，2019年突破200例，2020年开展SLT达387例，2015—2020年总共开展SLT 964例。2015—2020年各中心开展SLT例数排名依次为上海交通大学医学院附属仁济医院172例、天津市第一中心医院167例、中山大学附属第三医院133例、浙江大学医学院附属第一医院116例、四川大学华西医院67例。此外，值得注意的是，2018—2020年各年度SLT受者＜18岁例数分别为81例、139例和197例，超过受者总数50%，表明未成年人仍是SLT的主要对象。

SLT供肝根据获取方式可分为在体劈离和离体劈离两种，在体劈离实施手术时能够不阻断供肝血流，显著减少冷缺血时间，同时有利于辨认肝动、静脉及胆管等组织，减少肝断面出血及胆瘘等并发症，更合理的分配供肝血管，进而提高劈离供肝的质量，因此在国际上被广泛采用。

常规肝脏劈离方式包括经典劈离方式和完全左、右半肝劈离方式两种。将供肝劈离为左外叶（Ⅱ～Ⅲ段）和扩大的右三叶（Ⅰ+Ⅳ～Ⅷ段）的方式称为经典劈离，主要用于受者为儿童和成人的组合。将供肝劈离为左半肝（Ⅰ～Ⅳ段）和右半肝（Ⅴ～Ⅷ段）的方式称为完全左、右半肝劈离，用于体重匹配的 2 例成人受者。供肝完全劈离时应严格根据肝中静脉走行、解剖特点以及左右半肝体积等情况来决定肝中静脉的分配。浙江大学附属第一医院郑树森院士团队创新性采用异体冷保存的髂血管架桥重建肝静脉流出道，维持第Ⅴ段和第Ⅷ段的肝静脉回流，使得不含肝中静脉的右半肝活体肝移植及劈离式肝移植成为安全可靠的手术方式。

除了手术方式的日益改进，我国移植界对于供受体评估及匹配原则的认知也在逐渐完善。2020 年 10 月中华医学会外科学分会推出了我国第一版劈离式肝移植专家共识，进一步推动了 SLT 的规范化与标准化。SLT 与全肝移植的预后已十分相近，但其对于供受体的选择更为严格、准入标准更高，通常只限于肝脏体积、肝脏功能、年龄、血循环等诸方面条件均理想的供肝。目前，我国通常遵循以下供肝标准：①年龄小于 50 岁；②肝功能基本正常，没有或仅有轻度脂肪肝（＜10%）；③血流动力学稳定，无须大量血管活性药物的支持；④ ICU 时间少于 5 天；⑤血钠低于160mmol/L 等。

3. 小结

2015 年以来，我国开始全面进入公民逝世后器官捐献来源供肝时代，供肝短缺的形势仍然较为严峻。SLT 作为肝移植的成熟术式可有效扩大供肝来源，缩短受体等待时间。通过谨慎的供受体评估及熟练的 SLT 外科技术，能够显著提高 SLT 术后的疗效。在合理的器官分配政策下，通过多中心合作，我国将安全规范地推动 SLT的开展，更好地为人民服务。

六、低龄、低体重婴幼儿供肾成人肾脏移植的临床诊疗不断完善，获得良好临床效果

我国器官捐献率较发达国家低，捐献器官的相对缺乏仍是一个长期问题，而较之成人，我国的儿童监护人相对容易接受器官捐献理念，社会关系相对单纯，因此

儿童甚至婴儿器官捐献能在一定程度上扩大供体池，应得到进一步关注。婴儿供肾成人肾移植一般采用双肾整块移植方式，由于手术难度大，术后容易出现血管和输尿管并发症，国际最早报道于 20 世纪 70 年代。国内则最早报道于 1981 年，之后的 30 多年鲜有报道，因此开展此项手术的移植中心及病例数并不多。随着我国公民逝世后器官捐献工作的进展及外科技术的不断提高，在克服术中麻醉风险、改良供、受体血管吻合方式、精确处理术后抗凝 – 出血矛盾及重视术后并发症的防治等方面取得创新性进展后，近年来低龄、低体重（＜5kg）新生儿双供肾肾脏移植技术在一些医疗机构陆续开展。尽管目前例数较少，但已取得了可喜成果。华中科技大学同济医学院附属协和医院对 38 例低体重（＜5kg）婴儿双供肾成人肾脏移植进行了回顾性分析，结果显示移植肾 1 年存活率 76.3%，受者存活率 100%，相关研究发表于2021 年《中华器官移植杂志》上。

七、基于宏基因组学的二代测序技术在肾脏移植术后重症肺炎诊疗中的应用

肺部感染是肾脏移植术后受者最常见的感染及致死原因，尤其是多病原体混合感染的死亡率可达 50%，快速确定病原微生物是治疗的关键。临床常用的传统培养、革兰染色、免疫检测和核酸检测等方法，其时效性、敏感性和特异性不够理想，不利于重症感染的早期诊断与治疗。

基于宏基因组学的二代测序技术（metagenomic next-generation sequencing，mNGS）是新一代的病原微生物鉴定方式，在过去的 5 年经历了快速发展。该技术通过对临床样本中的核酸进行高通量测序，能够快速、客观的检测样本中的多种病原微生物（包括病毒、细菌、真菌和寄生虫等），尤其适用于急危重症和疑难感染的病原学诊断。由于 mNGS 具有检测速度快、准确率高、覆盖度广、检测结果受抗生素影响较小的优势，近年来国内一些大型医疗机构在常规检测基础上，将 mNGS 技术应用于肾脏移植术后重症肺炎的诊疗中，可在 24～48h 确定肺部感染病原体，对肾脏移植术后混合感染、肺孢子菌、巨细胞病毒感染导致的重症肺炎具有较好的诊断价值，有利于指导抗生素的临床应用，改善预后。相关研究已发表于 2021 年 *Ann Transplant* 和 *Bioengineered* 等期刊。

八、优化心脏移植围术期管理策略

心脏移植是治疗终末期心脏病最为有效的手段，面对我国庞大的心力衰竭患者群体与稀缺供体资源之间的矛盾，心力衰竭患者的规范化治疗、优化心脏移植受者规范化评估和筛选等措施是解决矛盾最主要的切入点。

不断提升心力衰竭规范化诊疗，使心力衰竭患者的病情进展得以延缓，把有限的供体资源供给最紧急及能获益最大的心力衰竭患者。

在围术期管理方面，大部分移植中心已形成多学科综合诊治的心衰与心脏移植治疗团队，探索了危重心力衰竭患者机械辅助桥接移植的最佳策略，完成国内最大组机械辅助（包括 ECMO、IABP 及 ECMO 联合 IABP 和左心辅助装置）过渡心脏移植的探索性应用和经验总结，建立了心脏移植前受体合并肺动脉高压评估及围术期处理方案，降低了危重患者等待期间的死亡率和心脏移植围术期死亡率，极大改善了心脏移植患者的短期和长期预后。

九、人工心脏的自主研制和临床应用

在心脏移植的替代治疗方面，我国已有三款具有自主知识产权的第三代全磁悬浮人工心脏在多中心开展临床试验。该类产品采用磁悬浮无接触轴承，体积小，生物相容性好，是世界上最先进的人工心脏之一。目前已经在中国医学科学院阜外医院、华中科技大学同济医学院附属协和医院完成了 25 例临床试验。

十、劈裂式肺叶移植

对于胸腔较小或是儿童患者来说，等待大小匹配的供肺难度极大，而肺叶移植可以解决此类问题并且术后效果与正常肺移植无明显差别。既往右肺劈裂式移植一般使用右上肺和右下肺分别给 1 名患者移植，右中肺为了避免中间段气管残端的出现往往选择舍弃。无锡市人民医院肺移植团队开创了全球首例劈裂式右上 / 中肺叶和右下肺叶移植，术中重建右上 / 中叶气管开口袖带进行吻合。此术式保留了右中叶，增加了患者术后的肺容积。另一方面，剪短中间段气管可减少右下肺无用腔，有利于气道的吻合和修复。气管镜检查及胸部影像学随访结果显示肺膨胀良好，无明显吻合并发症发生，表明该策略是安全可行的，且作为一种特殊的肺叶移植，值得在经验丰富的中心推广。该技术的详细病例报告 *A Modified Lobar Transplants Combining RUL and RML for Small Recipients* 已发表于美国《胸外科年鉴》（*Annals of Thoracic Surgery*）。

十一、异位肺移植

近年来，肺移植的发展受到供体来源缺乏的限制，尤其是全球新冠肺炎疫情影响，进一步加剧了供体短缺。随着肺移植气管吻合技术的发展，异位肺移植突破了供肺原位移植的桎梏，使得原本放弃的供肺可重新利用以挽救重症患者的生命。无锡市人民医院肺移植团队共完成 4 例异位肺移植，其中 3 例为单肺异位移植（1 例左供肺移植右胸腔，2 例右供肺移植左胸腔）。上述 3 例患者通过术中将一侧供肺沿上下轴旋转 180° 后植入对侧胸腔，供、受体支气管的膜部和软骨部交错吻合，供体的肺动脉沿肺动脉干充分游离，保留足够的长度以便顺延到支气管轴的前侧与受者肺动脉吻合，保证吻合时没有张力。肺静脉供、受体的房袖按照常规方法吻合。另一例为小胸腔女性患者完成的劈裂式双侧肺叶异位移植手术。供体右肺按解剖劈裂为右上肺和右中下肺。右上肺旋转后植入受体左侧胸腔而右中下肺植入右侧胸腔。所有手术均顺利完成；随访期间受体气管镜检查和胸部影像学结果显示移植肺扩张良好且随着时间的推移形态上能够适应并填满胸腔，证明了异位肺移植的安全性和可行性。

十二、心肺联合移植

对于终末期心肺功能衰竭患者而言，进行心肺联合移植是目前唯一有效的治疗手段。心肺联合移植的开展及推广受限主要是因为外科手术难度极高及相关的严重并发症，其中后纵隔出血尤为突出。广州医科大学附属第一医院肺移植团队针对此突出问题做出了努力与技术改进，创新发展了微异位式心肺联合移植术。传统心肺联合移植需要切除受体的隆凸及左右主支气管，然后供–受体的气管原位吻合。微异位式心肺联合移植术断离受体气管后，不再切除隆凸及左右主支气管，而是腔内处理后仍保留于受体体内，而供体气管叠在受体隆凸上与受体气管近端断端进行吻合。

该方法减少后纵隔切除范围，减少了手术出血特别是对于侧支循环丰富者更加明显，缩短了手术时间。该技术文章 *Non-In Situ Technique of Heart-Lung Transplantation: Case Series and Technique Description* 发表于美国《胸外科年鉴》(*Annals of Thoracic Surgery*)。

十三、创新性提出了潜在器官捐献者便捷评估方法

根据中国器官捐献国情，为了方便各级各类医院尤其是基层医院医务人员及时识别评估上报潜在器官捐献者，中国人民解放军南部战区总医院器官获取组织（GHOPO）创新性提出了潜在器官捐献者便捷评估方法，即 ABC-HOME。该方法将潜在器官捐献者年龄（age，A）、不可逆脑损伤和脑死亡（irreversible brain damage or brain death，B）、禁忌证（contradication，C）和循环情况（circulation，C）等归纳为 ABC，只要符合 ABC 即为可能的捐献者，进而将病史（history，H）、器官功能状况（organ function，O）、用药情况（medication，M）和内环境（internal environment，E）等归纳为 HOME，只要满足 ABC-HOME 的条件即为潜在器官捐献者。在此基础上如获得了潜在捐献者家属的知情同意，则为合格的器官捐献者。ABC-HOME 方法显著提高了潜在器官捐献者上报率，显著提高了 ICU 每张病床产生潜在器官捐献者的人数。

Report on Organ Transplantation Development in China (2020)

Editor-in-chief: Huang Jiefu

Compiled by China Organ Transplantation Development Foundation

China Science and Technology Press

· Beijing ·

Report on Organ Transplantation Development in China(2020) Editorial Committee

Preface

Organ transplantation is a major biomedical development in the 20th century. It has gradually matured from clinical experiments to clinical applications and has become an effective medical procedure for treating late-stage organ failure. It has saved thousands of patients with organ failure and promoted biomedical science development in China. As organ transplantation requires organs from either deceased or living-related donors, it involves social, religious, ethical, political, and legal issues, and is closely intertwined with a country's traditional culture and socioeconomic development.

Organ transplantation needs to comply with globally recognized code of ethics, take root in China's traditional culture, and match the state of social development in China. The Chinese government attaches great importance to the development of human organ donation and transplantation. On March 16, 2006, the then Ministry of Health issued the "Interim Provisions on Clinical Application and Management of Human Organ Transplantation" (MOH[1] [2006] No. 94), which clarified the requirements, promulgated technical norms, and regulated institutions' access to organ transplantation. In the same year, the National Human Organ Transplantation Clinical Application Management Summit was held in Guangzhou. Transplant professionals reached consensus and jointly issued the "Guangzhou Declaration". In May 2007, "Regulation on Human Organ Transplantation" (hereinafter referred to as "Regulation") was officially promulgated by the State Council of the People's Republic of China. This symbolized the start of legislative construction of human organ donation and transplantation system in China. In the same year, the then Ministry of Health issued the "Notice of the General Office of the Ministry of Health on the Issues Concerning the Application by Overseas Personnel for Human Organ Transplantation" (MOH [2007] No. 110) stipulating that foreign citizens are prohibited from coming to China with the purpose of receiving organ transplantation in the name of transplant tourism. In 2010, the then Ministry of Health and the Red Cross Society of China jointly initiated the "Pilot Program of Organ Donation from Citizens after Death". Based on the social development status and traditional culture, China established a human organ donation system within which the Red Cross Society of China participates as a third party. Meanwhile, according to international common practice and

---

1　MOH: Ministry of Health

China's national conditions, the Chinese professional community innovatively proposed the three types of Chinese criteria and procedures for voluntary organ donation after citizens' death: China Categories Ⅰ (C-Ⅰ, organ donation after brain death), Ⅱ (C-Ⅱ, organ donation after circulatory death), and Ⅲ (C- Ⅲ, organ donation after brain death followed by circulatory death). This laid the theoretical foundation for the deceased donation in China. In 2011, China promulgated the Amendment Ⅷ to the Criminal Law, adding "organ trafficking crime" to combat against crimes of organ trafficking, which further strengthened the legislation of organ donation. In terms of organ allocation, documents regulating the allocation principles in China were released in 2010. In 2011, the China Organ Transplant Response System (COTRS) was officially launched, which made scientific and equal allocation through computing system feasible. The organ donation coordinator team started to form in the same year.

On February 25th, 2013, based on pilot experiences, the nationwide deceased organ donation program was officially initiated jointly by the then Ministry of Health and the Red Cross Society of China. In August 2013, the then National Health and Family Planning Commission promulgated the "Interim Provisions on the Administration of Human Organ Procurement and Allocation", which requested the formal establishment of OPOs, designated service areas, clarified the mandatory use of COTRS by all transplant hospitals, and forbade organ allocation outside the COTRS by any institution, organization or individual, to ensure that donated human organs are allocated in an open, fair, equal, and traceable manner. On December 19th, 2013, the General Office of the Chinese Communist Party and the General Office of the State Council issued the "Opinions on Party Members and Cadres in Leading Funeral Reform" that encouraged party members and cadres to donate organs and cadavers after death. In March 2014, the Human Organ Transplantation Technology Clinical Application Committee (OTC) merged with the Human Organ Donation Committee to form the China Organ Donation and Transplantation Committee, which is responsible for the top-level design of the national organ transplantation in China. As the Chinese saying "It takes 10 years to forge a sword" goes, China has undergone reform, and gradually established the Chinese human organ donation and transplantation scheme, which is made up of 5 major components: human organ donation system, human organ procurement and allocation system, human organ transplantation medical service system, human organ procurement and transplantation quality control system, and the human organ donation and transplantation monitoring system. China has greatly promoted a loving spirit of organ donation in the whole society. A fair, transparent, and cheery atmosphere of voluntary organ donation by citizens has gradually formed. From January 1st, 2015, donation by citizens became the only legal source of organ for transplantation, marking the historic turning point of organ source in China.

Health is a common pursuit of mankind. Health of the whole world needs China's continuous efforts, while healthcare in China also requires support from the international community. In recent years, China has gradually strengthened communication and collaboration with other countries and comprehensively demonstrated the top-level design, system construction, laws and regulations and working system of organ transplantation in China. In addition, China has provided detailed data and analysis results to the international community through the World Health Organization Global Observatory on Organ Donation and Transplantation[2] to demonstrate China's achievements in human organ donation and transplantation reform in an open and transparent manner. With recognition and support from the international community, a set of articles on the reform were published in highly reputable international journals such as *the Lancet* and *Transplantation*. Many international experts have directly participated in and witnessed the process of China's organ transplantation reform and recognized the progress and improvements achieved by China. In August 2016, the 26th International Congress of The Transplantation Society was held in Hong Kong, the first TTS Annual Congress held in China. Professor Huang Jiefu delivered a keynote speech in the opening ceremony, and introduced China's 10–year organ transplantation reform journey to the world. In October 2016, the 1st "China-International Organ Donation Conference" (CIODC) was convened in the Gold Hall of the Great Hall of the People in Beijing. Renowned experts from transplantation societies overseas participated in the event and witnessed China's step towards the international community. In February 2017, China was invited to participate in the "Summit on Organ Trafficking and Transplant Tourism" organized by the Pontifical Academy of Sciences. During the summit, Chinese representatives presented China's voice and laid down the facts of China's transplant reform, which was highly praised by the world leaders. The "Chinese protocol" for organ donation and transplantation was recognized by the World Health Organization as China's innovation and contribution to the global development of organ donation and transplantation. During the event, Professor Francis Delmonico, chairman of the WHO

2　GODT, http://www.transplant-observatory.org/

Task Force on Donation and Transplantation of Human Organs and Tissues, mentioned that "Your bones are also our bones, your improvement is also our improvement", and welcomed China to the international transplantation community. Professor José Ramón Núñez, medical officer in charge of transplantation at World Health Organization once said that "China wasn't on the ship of world organ transplantation, and we had no idea where it was headed. But since 2015, China has been standing in the center of the ship." In March 2018, China's experience on facilitating the organ transplantation reform was included in the final declaration of the "Ethics in Action" meeting jointly organized by the United Nations and the Pontifical Academy of Sciences. The "Final Declaration of the Ethics in Action Meeting on Modern Slavery, Human Trafficking, and Access to Justice for the Poor and Vulnerable" mentioned that "An essential feature of the China Model is showing the resolution of the Chinese Government to sustain reform, effectively driven by the cooperation of professionals and exemplified the leadership of Professor Jiefu Huang." In May 2018, more than 100 Chinese transplant experts attended the side-event on organ transplantation of the 71st World Health Assembly, and introduced China's experience on advancing organ transplantation reforms. Dr. Tedros Adhanom, Director-General of the World Health Organization, praised and thanked China for its contribution to the development of organ transplantation across the world. In August 2018, the WHO Task Force on Donation and Transplantation of Human Organs and Tissues – which was proposed by China – was officially formed at the 27th International Congress of The Transplantation Society in Madrid, Spain. The Task Force gathered 31 experts; with Huang Jiefu being nominated as a World Health Organization transplantation advisor. China has started contributing its wisdom to global governance of transplantation.

In recent years, China has successively promulgated and established legislations and regulations to promote organ donation and transplantation. For example, in 2016, 6 ministries including the Ministry of Transport, Civil Aviation Administration of China, and then National Railway Administration, etc., jointly set up the green channel for organ transportation to win precious time to save lives. In May 2017, the "Law on the Red Cross Society of the People's Republic of China" was revised to stipulate the responsibility of the Red Cross Society on advancing the development of organ donation. The quantity and quality of organ donation and transplantation in China have undergone rapid development at the same time. From 2015 to 2018, the number of living-related organ donation in China remained stable (2200~2500 cases per year), while that of deceased organ donation showed significant increases. In 2015, 2016, 2017, and 2018, the number of deceased organ donation was 2766, 4080, 5146, and 6302, respectively. In 2018, with 20 201 cases of organ transplantation performed, China ranked the second globally. Since 2019, China's organ donation and transplantation started its shift from high-speed growth to high-quality development. With a purpose of achieving high quality, more efficient, more equitable and sustainable development, China will adhere to the supply-side structural reform, put emphasis on the optimization of the layout of organ transplantation clinical services, while vigorously enhance the level of quality of organ donation. Administration on organ donation, organ procurement and allocation will also be strengthened to achieve a quantitative growth with excellent quality. In 2019, 5818 cases of deceased organ donation were completed. In 2020, despite of the influence of the COVID-19 pandemic, China still saw 5222 cases of deceased organ donation. In addition, quality of organ transplants in China has also been constantly improved. The 1-year and 5-year survival rates of China are among the top in the world. Innovative technologies are also emerging. For example, China is at the frontier of autologous liver transplantation and non-ischemic organ transplantation; breakthroughs have been achieved in incompatible blood type kidney transplantation; clinical capabilities of pediatric liver transplantation, heart transplantation, and lung transplantation of single center are in the forefront of the world; continuous improvements have been made in organ preservation and maintenance technology. China's clinical experience in liver cancer liver transplantation and hepatitis B liver transplantation have also received international recognition. After years of efforts, a scientific, fair, and ethical working model based on China's social and cultural reality has been established, the basic thought on human organ donation and transplantation has been formed, a "government-led, department-coordinated, industry-promoted, and society-supported" working structure has been achieved.

In October 2019, the Fourth Plenary Session of the 19th Central Committee of the Chinese Communist Party stressed the request on upholding and improving the system of socialism with Chinese characteristic, promoting the construction of national governance system and advancing the modernization of governance capabilities. On May 28th, 2020, the Civil Code of the People's Republic of China was officially promulgated. Chapter 4 (Personality Rights) of the Civil Code protects citizen's right for voluntary organ donation, while strictly prohibits human organ trafficking. "It takes a good blacksmith to make steel" – the new era puts forward higher requirements for organ transplantation. We will actively heed the call of the party, advance modernization in organ transplantation reform, strengthen system and capacity building, face challenges in a bold and steadfast manner, and continuously improve ourselves to protect achievements that were not easily obtained. We will strive to establish a complete organ donation and transplantation system that complies with ethics and principles of the World Health Organization, strive to reach the science and medical peaks in organ transplantation, actively promote international collaboration in organ donation and transplantation under the framework of "Belt and Road Initiative", and contribute to the construction of "community with a shared future for mankind".

This Report documents the achievements of the new stage in the history of organ transplantation, and will show the world the experience and achievements of organ transplantation reform in China. The China Organ Transplant Development Foundation will organize the compilation and publication of the Report every year, in both Chinese and English.

Editorial Committee

August, 2021

Contents

Chapter 1 Organ Procurement in China

1.1 Development of Organ Procurement Organization in China

As the development cornerstone and bridge connecting organ donation and transplantation, Organ Procurement Organization (OPO) in China emerged with the launch of the citizens' voluntary organ donation system. OPOs are composed of professionals dedicated to the work in the whole process of organ procurement and allocation. Surgeons, neurologists, neurosurgeons, critical care physicians and nurses, as well as human organ donation coordinators are the core members of OPO. OPOs are professional organizations engaged in the donation and procurement of human organs after the death of citizens. The OPO teams are officially selected and formed by the provincial health authorities. Major responsibilities of OPOs include: organ donation related public education; donor information collection; potential donor identification, evaluation, maintenance and referral; organ procurement, recovery, allocation, transportation; as well as dealing with the matters after organ donation and commemorating the organ donors.

On August 13th, 2013, the then National Health and Family Planning Commission released the *Interim Provisions on the Administration of Human Organ Procurement and Allocation* (NHFPC[1]〔2013〕No. 11), which required the use of ethical organs from deceased donors; the selection and formation of OPOs and the establishment of professional coordinator teams on human organ donation; the clarification of service areas of OPOs; and the mandatory use of the China Organ Transplant Response System (COTRS) for all donated organs, with the purpose of establishing a fair, transparent and traceable organ procurement and allocation system. This document symbolized a new era, starting from which OPOs started to step on to the historical stage of organ donation and transplantation in China.

Another official document named *Notice on Strengthening Administration of Donated Organ Procurement and Allocation* (NHFPC〔2013〕No. 16), was released on September 3rd, 2013, by the then National Health and Family Planning Commission. This document authorized the provincial health administrative institutions with the responsibility of supervising and planning the development of OPOs within the province, and provided guidance on zoning, establishment, and change of the

---

1 NHFPC: National Health and Family Planning Commission

service areas of OPOs. On March 20th, 2014, the Association of Organ Procurement Organizations, Chinese Hospital Association was launched. This marked the formal management of OPOs in China, setting the basis for standardized management and self-discipline in organ transplantation. On December 3rd, 2014, at the Organ Procurement Organization (OPO) Alliance Conference, Huang Jiefu, Chairman of the China Human Organ Donation and Transplantation Committee, announced that from January 1st, 2015, voluntary donation from citizens became the only legal source of organ for transplantation in China, which signified that China's organ transplantation has entered a new development stage.

On October 16th, 2016, on the basis of the OPO Alliance, Chinese Hospital Association initiated the Organ Procurement and Allocation Administrative Committee of Chinese Hospital Association (CHA-COPO), which marked a new development era for OPOs in China. The CHA-COPO was supervised and guided by the Bureau of Medical Administration, National Health Commission and the China Human Organ Donation and Transplantation Commission, and was charged with the responsibility regarding the construction of organ procurement and allocation system of the China Organ Donation and Transplant Scheme.

Entrusted by the National Health and Family Planning Commission and China Human Organ Donation and Transplantation Commission, based on previous works, CHA-COPO published a set of regulations: the *Interim Provisions on the Cost Accounting and Financial Management of Human Organ Procurement and Transplantation (Draft)* was published on January 1st, 2017, which was an important reference for OPOs across the country to gradually establish the standardized cost accounting and financial management system. The *Administrative Provisions for Organ Procurement Organizations* was accepted by the National Health Commission. Based on a nationwide consultation, it developed into the *Administrative Regulation on Donated Organ Procurement and Allocation* (NHC[2] [2019] No. 2), formally released by the National Health Commission on January 17th, 2019. Another important document was the *Basic Requirements and Quality Control Indicators of Organ Procurement Organizations* released by the National Health Commission in February 2019. Purposes of this document were to regulate the construction and development of OPOs and to establish a quality management and control system for OPOs. This document has adopted and revised the *OPO Quality Control Standards* (originally drafted by the CHA-COPO), clarified 9 quality control indicators regarding the construction of OPO, specified fundamental requirements, including general management requirements, human resource requirements and technical requirements of medical institutions with OPOs. This documents thus played an important role in regulating the management of Organ Procurement Organizations in China.

2　NHC: National Health Commission

1.2 Distribution of OPOs

In 2020, there were 133 OPOs in China. Provinces that have established provincial unified OPOs were Shanxi, Jilin, Tianjin, and Hainan. Provinces that have built joint OPO management systems were Guangdong, Beijing, Hunan, Shanghai, Hebei and Fujian (Figure 1–1).

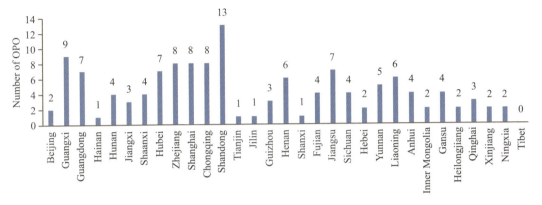

▲ **Figure 1–1   Number of OPOs by provinces (autonomous regions and cities) in 2020**

1.3 Organ Donation in China

In 2020, the 10 provinces (autonomous regions, cities) with the most cases of organ donation were: Guangdong (818), Beijing (496), Shandong (390), Hunan (373), Guangxi (356), Henan (309), Zhejiang (280), Hubei (278), Jiangxi (250) and Shaanxi (202). Number of donors per million population (PMP) of 14 provinces (autonomous regions, cities) has surpassed the national average level (3.70). The 10 provinces (autonomous regions, cities) with the highest PMP were: Beijing (22.66), Guangxi (7.10), Guangdong (6.49), Hainan (6.05), Hunan (5.61), Jiangxi (5.53), Shaanxi (4.81), Hubei (4.81), Zhejiang (4.34), and Shanghai (4.02) (Figure 1–2).

1.4 Organs generated per donor

In 2020, the average number of organs generated per donor in China was 3.14. The average number of livers generated per donor was 0.94, that of kidneys was 1.90, that of hearts were 0.11, and that of lungs were 0.18 (Figure 1–3 to Figure 1–7).

Among the 75 OPOs with more than 20 organ donation cases annually, the 10 OPOs with the greatest of number of organs generated per donor were: Joint OPO of Southern Beijing District (4.21), The First Affiliated Hospital of Guangzhou Medical University (4.07), The First Affiliated Hospital of Soochow University (3.72), Joint OPO of Northern Beijing District (3.71), The Second Affiliated Hospital of Guangzhou Medical University (3.7), The Second Affiliated Hospital, Zhejiang University School of Medicine (3.6), Guangdong Provincial People's Hospital (3.6), The Affiliated Hospital of

Qingdao University (3.47), The Seventh People's Hospital of Zhengzhou (3.46), Tianjin First Central Hospital (3.46).

1.5 Quality Control of Donated Organ Procurement

The three major components of donated organ procurement quality control are organizational quality control of OPOs, quality control of donors, and quality control of organs procured.

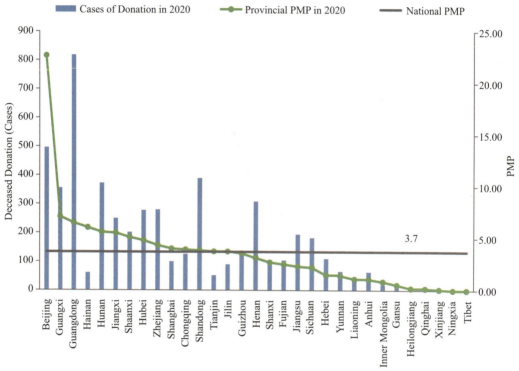

▲ **Figure 1−2**　**Number of organs donated and PMP by provinces (autonomous regions and cities) in 2020**

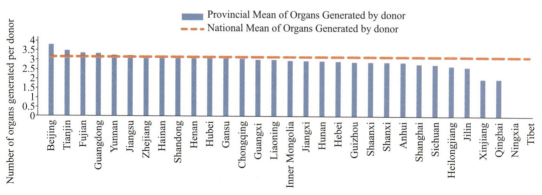

▲ **Figure 1−3**　**Organs generated per donor by provinces (autonomous regions and cities)**

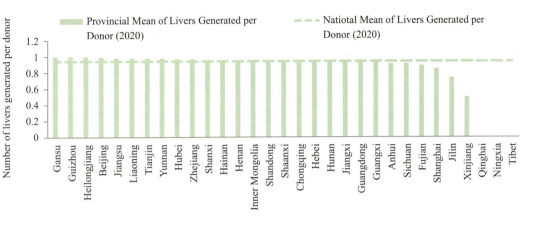

▲ Figure 1-4   Livers generated per donor by provinces (autonomous regions and cities)

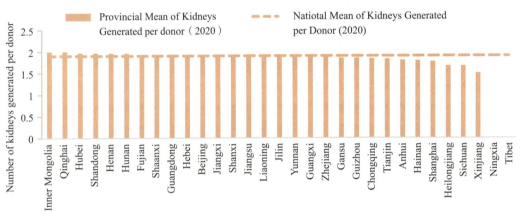

▲ Figure 1-5   Kidneys generated per donor by provinces (autonomous regions and cities)

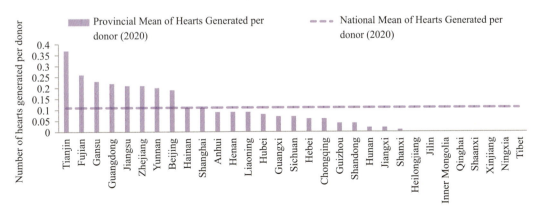

▲ Figure 1-6   Hearts generated per donor by provinces (autonomous regions and cities)

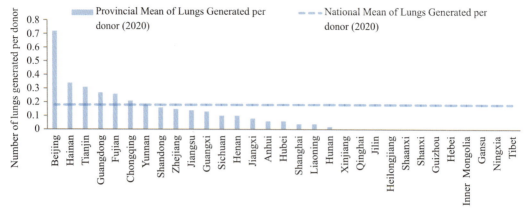

▲ **Figure 1-7**　**Lungs generated per donor by provinces (autonomous regions and cities)**

1.5.1　Organizational quality control of OPOs

From the perspective of the construction of OPOs, it is essential to strengthen the quality control from 3 aspects including regulated operation, performance measurement, and technical development. 29 indicators were proposed for OPO Quality Control and Management, including 9 core indicators, 9 performance indicators, 6 technical indicators and 5 reference indicators. Among the 29 indicators, 9 have been formally released by the National Health Commission: organ donor conversion rate, proportional distribution of organ donor categories, average number of organs generated per donor; organ use rate[3], percentage of marginal grafts, organ pathological examination rate, positive rate of bacterial culture in the organ preservation solutions, primary non-functioning rate of transplanted organs, rate of delayed graft function after transplantation.

1.5.2　Quality control of donors

Quality control of donors includes the confirmation and evaluation of medical history, clinical situation, vasoactive drug use dosage, laboratory test results, tumor screening, infection screening, and organ puncture pathological evaluation. OPOs could provide quality control services to transplant centers by the above measures.

1.5.3　Quality control of organs procured

Quality control of organs procured includes the evaluation of the morphology, anatomy, and damage of the donor liver, kidney, heart, lung, pancreas, etc.

1.6　Features and Prospects

Supported by the central government of China and directly supervised by the National

---

3　Carámbula A, Mizraji R, Godino M, Castro A, Bengochea M. Organ Use Rate: A New Indicator of Donation and Transplantation Efficiency. Transplant Proc. 2020;52(4):1070-1071. doi:10.1016/ j.transproceed.2020.02.016

Health Commission and the Red Cross Society of China, the China Human Organ Donation and Transplantation Committee has been committed to unifying all related parties, and has successfully established the "Chinese Model" of organ donation and transplantation based on strict compliance with the international codes of ethics. We have realized the successful transition of human organ sources. Furthermore, to fully protect the rights and interests of organ donors and transplant recipients, a fair and traceable organ allocation system has been set up over the past years. In order to further consolidate the healthy and sustainable development of organ donation and transplantation in China, we have to devote ourselves to establishing and advancing the OPOs based on the "Chinese Model" and the reality of China. To further promote the development of organ procurement, emphasis should be put on the following aspects.

1.6.1 Regulating the management of OPOs

To enhance the quality of OPOs, it is essential to regulate and standardize the organizational structure, personnel structure, job responsibilities, and operation procedures. Effective process control and supervision should also be considered and implemented. According to the *Administrative Regulation on Donated Organ Procurement and Allocation* (NHC〔2019〕No. 2), taking into consideration of the Chinese reality and current working basis, the next key direction should be: firstly, to set up and gradually unify OPOs on the premise of meeting people's medical needs in accordance with the plan of the provincial health authorities; secondly, ensure that OPOs conduct organ donation and procurement related activities in the designated service areas in a standardized manner.

1.6.2 Regulating the performance assessment and quality control of OPOs

With the establishment of the system of organ donation from citizens after death, organ transplantation in China is continually developing in a legal, ethical, and international way. This has also promoted the rise and construction of OPOs in China. The healthy development of China's deceased donation system relies on the systematic construction of OPO. Systems for donor identification, death diagnosis, donor organ maintenance, quality optimization, quality evaluation, research and regulation on organ procurement techniques should be established accordingly. These are closely related to the quality of donors and donated organs. Therefore, it is urgent to formulate donor and organ quality control standards, strictly control the quality of donors and donated organs, and provide high-quality medical services for patients with end-stage organ failure.

1.6.3 Establishing a unified quality control mechanism of organ procurement and allocation

We must improve the reporting of donor evaluation results, donor quality assessment results, infection and pathological examination results, establish an effective and standardized data sharing system, to enhance the unified quality control on organ allocation between OPOs and transplant hospitals, decrease discard rate of donated organs, reduce organ loss, thus save more patients with organ failure.

1.6.4 Establishing financial management mechanism in OPOs

In order to facilitate the healthy development of human organ procurement, it is important to calculate the organ procurement related costs in a standardized and transparent way. Therefore, organ procurement related charging policies should be established within each provincial jurisdiction to promote the well-regulated financial management of OPOs. Complete, standardized, and reasonable charging standards on organ procurement surgeries, recovery, maintenance, storage, transportation, examination, allocation, and transplantation should be set up.

Chapter 2 Human Organ Allocation and Sharing in China

The data showed in this chapter are mainly based on data analysis from the China Organ Transplant Response System (COTRS). The statistics represent that of the Mainland China, not including Hong Kong, Macao, and Taiwan regions of Peoples' Republic of China.

From January 1st, 2015 to December 31st, 2020, a total of 29,334 cases of organ donation after death (Deceased Donation, DD) have been completed in China. In 2020, 5222 deceased donations and 17 897 organ transplants were completed. The organ donation rate (per million population, PMP) increased from 2.01 in 2015 to 3.70 in 2020.

The Chinese human organ donation and transplantation scheme is consisted of 5 major components: human organ donation system, human organ procurement and allocation system, human organ transplantation medical service system, human organ procurement and transplantation quality control system, and the human organ donation and transplantation monitoring system (Figure 2−1), based on which China has established scientific, fair, and just organs allocation.

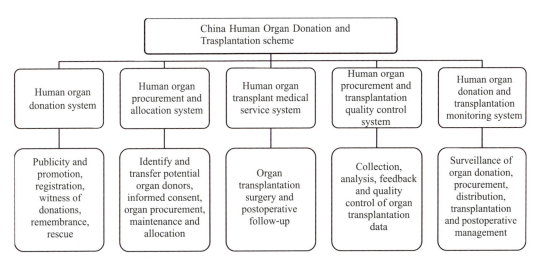

▲ Figure 2−1 China human organ donation and transplantation scheme (not including Hong Kong, Macao, and Taiwan regions)

COTRS is an important manifestation and implementation of legal provisions related to organ transplantation and donation in Articles 6 and 22 of the *"Regulation on Human Organ Transplantation"* and Article 234 of the *"Amendment Ⅷ to the Criminal Law"*. In 2018, the National Health Commission issued the *"Notice on Issuing the Basic Principles and Core Policies for the Allocation and Sharing of Human Organs in China"* (NHC〔2018〕No. 24), which revised the *"Notice of the Ministry of Health on Issuing the Basic Principles and Core Policies for the Allocation and Sharing of Human Organs for Liver and Kidney Transplantation"* (MOH-BMA[4]〔2010〕No. 113), and officially developed the core policies for the allocation and sharing of hearts and lungs. These combined formulated the *"Basic Principles and Core Policies for the Allocation and Sharing of Human Organs in China"* (Hereinafter referred to as the core policy of organ allocation).

China's organ allocation core policy is established in accordance with the principles and standards stipulated in the *"Regulation on Human Organ Transplantation"* promulgated by the State Council. It conforms to the international standards required by the World Health Organization and has incorporated Chinese characteristics. For example, to encourage citizens to donate organs after deaths, the immediate relatives, spouses, and collateral blood relatives of organ donors within the same geographical allocation area, or those who have been registered as Chinese organ donation volunteers for more than 3 years, will be given priority ranking in the allocation system. Meanwhile, living organ donors who need organ transplant surgery are also given priority in ranking.

COTRS is an essential part of China's organ donation and transplantation system, which is consists of "potential organ donor identification system", "human organ donor registration and organ matching system", "human organ transplant waiting list system" and the regulatory platform.

As a highly specialized system, COTRS is responsible for implementing the relevant laws, regulations, and scientific policies of organ allocation and sharing in China. It enforces the national policy for scientific organ allocation, enables automatic organ allocation and sharing, provides monitoring on national and local regulatory agencies, ensures the traceability of organ procurement and allocation, minimizes human interference, and guarantees the fair, just, and equitable allocation of donated organs. The COTRS system is managed by the China Organ Transplant Development Foundation.

2.1 Distribution of medical resources for organ donation and transplantation

2.1.1 Distribution of OPOs in China

In the system of human organ donation and transplantation in China, Organ Procurement Organization (OPO) is the professional team affiliated to medical institutions, entirely dedicated to organ donation and procurement. Different from the OPOs in the United States and the Organization

---

4   MOH-BMA: Ministry of Health, Bureau of Medical Administration

National De Transplants (ONT) in Spain, OPOs in China are composed of professional teams of medical personnel, organ donation coordinators, and administrative staff.

As of December 31st, 2020, there were 133 OPOs in China (not including Hong Kong, Macao, and Taiwan regions).

2.1.2 Distribution of transplant centers in China

As of December 31st, 2020, excluding Hong Kong, Macao, and Taiwan regions, there were 170 medical institutions qualified for organ transplantation in China. The distribution of these institutions by provinces (autonomous regions and cities) is shown in Figure 2–2. The ten provinces (autonomous regions and cities) with the greatest number of transplant centers were Guangdong (19), Beijing (17), Shandong (12), Shanghai (11), Hunan (9), Zhejiang (9), Fujian (8), Hubei (7), Guangxi (6), Henan (6), and Liaoning (6).

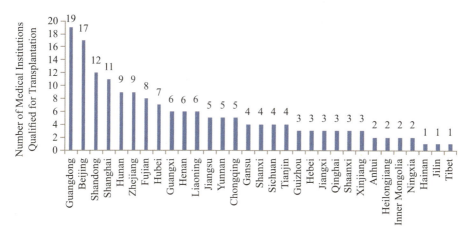

▲ Figure 2–2 Distribution of qualified medical institutions in China, 2020 (not including Hong Kong, Macao, and Taiwan regions)

2.2 Human Organ donation

2.2.1 Organ donation in China

From 2015 to 2020, the numbers of DD in Chinese citizens were 2766, 4080, 5146, 6302, 5818 and 5222, and PMPs were 2.01, 2.98, 3.72, 4.53, 4.16, 3.70, respectively (Figure 2–3).

In 2020, under the grim situation swept by the COVID-19 pandemic, Chinese organ donation and transplantation practitioners faced the difficulties and moved forward firmly to save patients with end-stage organ failure. As the COVID-19 pandemic in China eased since April 2020, organ donation work has resumed rapidly. Since June 2020, the amount of organ donation after the death of citizens has returned to the level of the same period in 2019 (Figure 2–4).

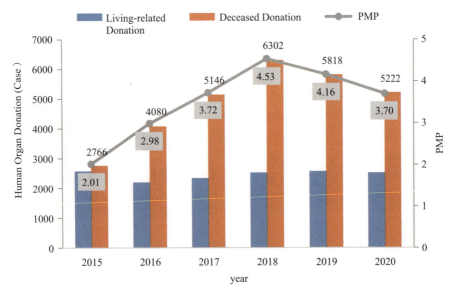

▲ **Figure 2–3 Numbers of Organ Donations in China (not including Hong Kong, Macao, and Taiwan regions)**

Data of population from 2015 to 2019 is obtained from the *China Health Statistics Yearbook*. Data of population in 2020 is obtained from National Bureau of Statistics of China

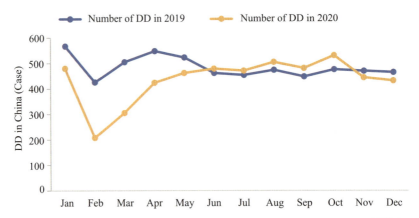

▲ **Figure 2–4 Trends in the number of human organ donations in China in 2020 (not including Hong Kong, Macao, and Taiwan regions)**

2.2.2 Characteristics of deceased donors

In 2020, the median age of DDs in China was 47. The number of pediatric donation (donors below the age of 18) was 413, accounting for 7.91% of the total. Among them, 81 donors (19.61%) were <2 years old, 99 donors (23.97%) were 2–6 years old, 117 (28.33%) were donors aged 7–13, and 116 (28.09%) were donors aged 14–17. The majority of donors was male (80.89%). The dominating (37.03%) blood type of the donors was Type O, followed by Type A and Type B, each accounting for 27.75% and 27.08% of all donors; Type AB accounted for 8.14% (Figure 2–5). 44.33% of DDs were C-I (donors after brain death ,DBD), 39.26% of DDs were C-Ⅱ (donors after circulatory death, DCD), 16.41% of DDs were C-Ⅲ (donors after brain death followed by cardiac death, DBCD) (Figure 2–6).

From 2015 to 2020, trauma and cerebrovascular accidents were two of the main causes of donors' death, accounting for 86.98% of all deaths (Figure 2–7). The proportion of donors with cerebrovascular accidents had been increasing each year. From 2019, cerebrovascular accidents have overtaken trauma as the leading cause of deaths in DDs in China (Figure 2–8).

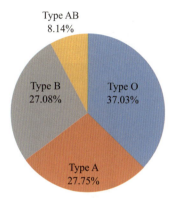

▲ Figure 2–5 Distribution of blood types of DDs in 2020 (not including Hong Kong, Macao, and Taiwan regions)

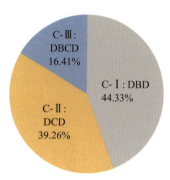

▲ Figure 2–6 Categories of DDs in 2020 (not including Hong Kong, Macao, and Taiwan regions)

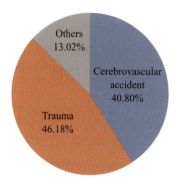

▲ Figure 2–7 Causes of DDs death, 2015–2020 (not including Hong Kong, Macao, and Taiwan regions)

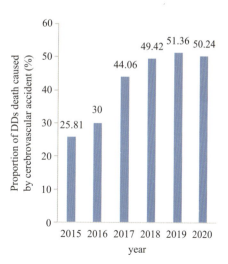

▲ Figure 2–8 Proportion of DDs death caused by cerebrovascular accident, 2015—2020 (not including Hong Kong, Macao, and Taiwan regions)

2.3 Patients waiting for organ transplantation

From 2015 to 2020, the number of patients waiting for liver and kidney transplantation had been increasing each year (Figure 2–9). In 2020, there were 96 550 people actively waiting for liver and kidney heart and lung transplants in China, including 78 324 waiting for kidney transplantation, 15 991 waiting for liver transplantation, 1423 waiting for heart transplantation, and 812 waiting for lung transplantation. During the same period, a total of 17 897 people (18.54%) received organ transplants across the country.

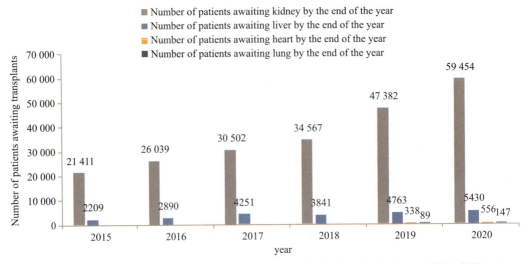

▲ **Figure 2–9** **Number of patients awaiting organ transplantation by the end of each year, 2015—2020 (not including Hong Kong, Macao, and Taiwan regions)**

By the end of 2020, there were 59 454 patients waiting for kidney transplantation and 5430 patients waiting for liver transplantation. The allocation system for heart and lung was initiated on October 22, 2018. By the end of 2020, there were still 556 and 147 patients waiting for heart and lung transplantation, respectively.

Figure 2–10 shows the numbers of patients waiting for kidney transplantation in each province (autonomous regions and cities) excluding Hong Kong, Macao, and Taiwan at the end of 2020. The top 10 provinces (autonomous regions and cities) were: Guangdong (7630), Zhejiang (5875), Hunan (5682), Sichuan (4949), Shanghai (4318), Hubei (4141), Henan (3041), Tianjin (2788), Shandong (2609), and Guangxi (2376).

Figure 2–11 shows the numbers of patients waiting for liver transplantation in each province (autonomous regions and cities) excluding Hong Kong, Macao, and Taiwan at the end of 2020. The top 10 provinces (autonomous regions and cities) were: Sichuan (1240), Guangdong (810), Tianjin (656), Shanghai (411), Zhejiang (365), Beijing (296), Hubei (256), Hunan (227), Jiangsu (154), and Yunnan (150).

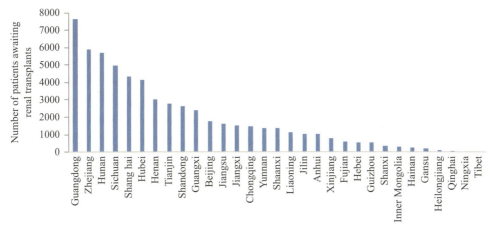

▲ **Figure 2-10**　**Numbers of patients awaiting kidney transplantation at the end of 2020 (not including Hong Kong, Macao, and Taiwan regions)**

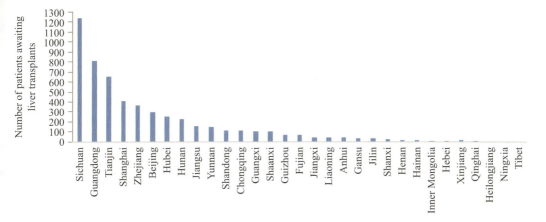

▲ **Figure 2-11**　**Numbers of patients awaiting liver transplantation at the end of 2020 (not including Hong Kong, Macao, and Taiwan regions)**

Figure 2-12 shows the numbers of patients waiting for heart transplantation in each province (autonomous regions and cities) excluding Hong Kong, Macao, and Taiwan at the end of 2020. The top 10 provinces (autonomous regions and cities) were: Beijing (154), Guangdong (69), Shanghai (60), Hubei (53), Henan (33), Zhejiang (33), Shandong (30), Hunan (27), Jiangsu (25), and Tianjin (14).

Figure 2-13 shows the numbers of patients waiting for lung transplantation in each province (autonomous regions and cities) excluding Hong Kong, Macao, and Taiwan at the end of 2020. The top 10 provinces (autonomous regions and cities) were: Jiangsu (29), Guangdong (28), Zhejiang (25), Henan (11), Hubei (10), Anhui (9), Sichuan (9), Beijing (8), Shanghai (8), and Hunan (5).

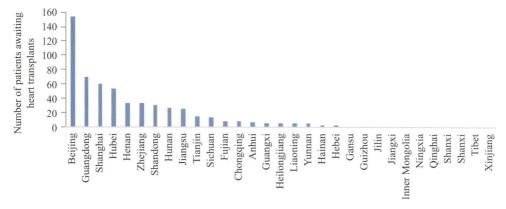

▲ **Figure 2−12** **Numbers of patients waiting for heart transplantation at the end of 2020(not including Hong Kong, Macao, and Taiwan regions)**

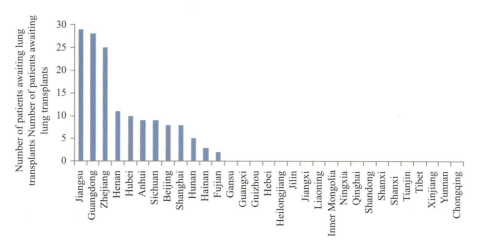

▲ **Figure 2−13** **Numbers of patients awaiting lung transplantation at the end of 2020 (not including Hong Kong, Macao, and Taiwan regions)**

2.4 Utilization of donated organ

2.4.1 Organs generated per donor

From 2015 to 2020, the average number of kidneys generated per donor after death were 1.92, 1.87, 1.89, 1.91, 1.89, and 1.90, and the average number of livers generated per donor were 0.88, 0.87, 0.90, 0.91, 0.93, and 0.94, respectively (Figure 2−14). In 2020, the average number of hearts generated per donor was 0.11, and the average number of lungs generated per donor was 0.18. Since the formulation of the core policy for the allocation of heart and lung in 2018, the number of hearts and lungs generated has increased year by year. Compared with 2019, the average number of lungs generated per donor has increased by 20% in 2020.

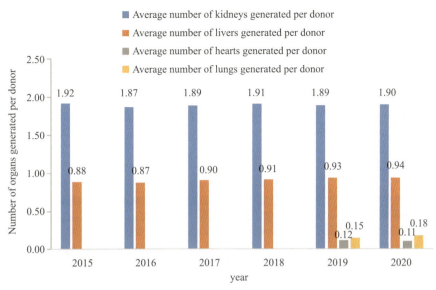

▲ Figure 2−14 **Average numbers of organs generated per donor 2015−2020 (not including Hong Kong, Macao, and Taiwan regions)**

2.4.2 Comparison of pediatric kidney transplantation before and after the revision of the organ allocation policy

The core organ distribution policy revised by the National Health Commission in 2018 further promotes and implements the principle of giving priority to protecting children's interests and promoting the allocation of public resources to children during the "13th Five-Year Plan" period. Considering the serious adverse effects of kidney disease and dialysis treatment on the growth and development of children, kidneys from donors under the age of 18 are allocated to kidney transplant waiters under 18 in priority nationwide, increasing the chance of getting donated kidney among children waiting for transplantation.

Comparing children's kidney transplants before and after the revision of the core organ distribution policy, the proportion of children receiving organs among the kidney transplant waiters rose from 2% to 3%, an increase of 50%.

2.4.3 Comparison of organ sharing before and after the implementation of the green channel policy

On May 6th, 2016, the then National Health and Family Planning Commission, the Ministry of Public Security, the Ministry of Transport, the Civil Aviation Administration of China, the then China Railway Corporation, and the China Red Cross Society jointly issued the *"Notice Regarding the Establishment of a Green Channel for the Transport of Human Donated Organs"* (hereinafter referred to as the "*Notice*") to establish a green channel for the transportation of human organs donated. The *Notice* clarifies the responsibilities of all parties to ensure the smooth transit of human donated organs and minimize the impact of transit on the quality and safety of organ transplantation.

The "*Notice*" categorized organ transit into general and emergency processes according to the specific situations to achieve a fast custom clearance and priority transportation of human donated organs, thus improve the efficiency and safety of the transits, as well as reduce the waste of organs caused by transportation.

Comparing the national sharing of human organs before and after the implementation of the *Green Channel Policy for Transport of Human Donated Organs*, the national rate of organ sharing has increased by 5.8%, of which the sharing of kidneys increased by 5.9%, and the sharing of livers increased by 3.9% (Table 2–1).

Table 2-1 Sharing of kidneys and livers in China before and after the implementation of the Green Channel Policy (not including Hong Kong, Macao, and Taiwan regions)									
Period	**Overall Sharing Rate（%）**			**Kidney Sharing Rate（%）**			**Liver Sharing Rate（%）**		
	Pre-policy	**Post-policy**	**Change**	**Pre-policy**	**Post-policy**	**Change**	**Pre-policy**	**Post-policy**	**Change**
Within transplant center	75.0	67.4	–7.6	84.6	75.9	–8.7	53.2	49.9	–3.3
Provincial level sharing	12.6	14.4	1.8	10.5	13.3	2.8	17.3	16.7	–0.6
National level sharing	12.4	18.2	5.8	4.9	10.8	5.9	29.5	33.4	3.9

2.5 Features and prospects

Organ transplantation is a great achievement in the development of human medicine, saving lives of countless patients with end-stage diseases. In 2020, the number of organ donations and transplants in China ranks the second in the world. COTRS is a highly specialized system for regulations and policies of organ allocation and sharing. It implements the national-level scientific allocation policy to ensure the fairness, justice and openness of organ allocation. However, it still faces issues that need to be resolved.

2.5.1 The scientific policy of organ allocation shall be updated regularly

The quality of organ allocation influenced by the biological matching of organs and recipients. The efficiency of organ allocation and sharing determines the quality of organs and the efficiency of organ utilization, which directly affects the survival rate and quality of life of transplant recipients.

In the next step, the China will establish the COTRS Scientific Committee, whose members will be composed of administrators and experts across the country. A regular working schedule will be established, to strengthen the research on scientific policymaking regarding organ allocation, focusing on improving the quality of organ matching, improving the efficiency of organ allocation, and reducing the mortality rate of patients waiting for organs. In addition, allocation policies of pancreas and small intestine will also be studied and promoted, providing more evidence for decision-making to the government.

2.5.2 Strengthen information feedback and promote continuous improvement of the quality of organ allocation

After over ten years of endeavor, China has gradually established a fair, just, and open human organ donation and allocation system, and formed a supervision and management mechanism featuring "informatization, government leadership, professional autonomy, and hospital self-inspection". Meanwhile, an information-based surveillance platform supported by big data has been established to trace the process from organ donation, procurement, allocation, to transplantation.

It is necessary to strengthen the dynamic monitoring of the quality of organ allocation; continue to provide feedback for the improvement of relevant indicators to various institutions including OPOs, medical institutions and health authorities; improve the degree of homogeneity of organ allocation quality among different medical institutions; reduce quality differences; and provide more efficient and scientific organ allocation.

Chapter 3 Liver Transplantation in China

The data showed in this chapter are mainly based on data analysis from the China Liver Transplant Registry(CLTR). Data of Hong Kong, Macao, and Taiwan regions were not included.

CLTR is the official registry system established by the National Health Committee of China. All transplant centers qualified for liver transplants are requested to report all the information related to the transplantation surgery in a timely and complete manner. CLTR conducts a dynamic and scientific analysis of liver transplantations in Mainland China, describes the medical quality status, hence provides policy-making basis for the administrative authorities. CLTR has also provided a scientific management tool of liver transplantation recipients for the transplant centers across China. As of now, CLTR has become one of the most important information systems and academic exchange platforms for liver transplantation in China.

3.1 Distribution of medical institutions qualified for liver transplantation

By December 31st, 2020, a total of 103 medical institutions were qualified to perform liver transplants. The top 10 provinces (autonomous regions and cities) with the greatest number of liver transplant centers were Beijing (12), Guangdong (12), Shanghai (9), Shandong (8), Zhejiang (6), Fujian (5), Guangxi (5), Hubei (5), Hunan (4), and Chongqing (4) (Figure 3–1).

From 2015 to 2020, 29 732 liver transplants have been performed, including 25 584 cases of Deceased Donor Liver Transplantation (DDLT) (86%) and 4,148 cases of Living-related Donor Liver Transplantation (LDLT) (14.0%) (Figure 3–2). There were 24 423 adult liver transplantations (82.1%) and 5309 pediatric liver transplantations (17.9%).

In 2020, 5842 liver transplantation were performed across the country, including 4,954 cases of DDLT (84.8%) and 888 cases of LDLT (15.2%), among which 14 cases were domino liver transplants and 5 cases were transplantation of discarded livers. There were 4663 cases of adult liver transplantation (79.8%), and 1179 cases of pediatric liver transplantation (20.2%). The 10 provinces (autonomous regions and cities) with the most liver transplants performed in 2020 were Shanghai (1172), Zhejiang (810), Guangdong (684), Beijing (556), Hunan (270), Tianjin (245), Henan (220), Jiangsu (197), Shandong (194), and Jiangxi (180). 16 provinces performed more than 100 liver transplants in 2020; the total amount of liver transplants performed in these provinces accounted for

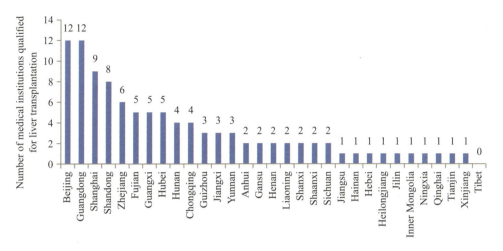

▲ **Figure 3-1** **Distribution of medical institutions qualified for liver transplantation in China in 2020 (not including Hong Kong, Macao, and Taiwan regions)**

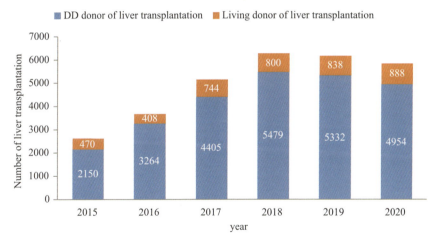

▲ **Figure 3-2** **Number of liver transplantation cases in China from 2015 to 2020 (not including Hong Kong, Macao, and Taiwan regions)**

92.4% of all cases in China (Figure 3-3). No liver transplant was performed in Ningxia and Qinghai. There were no medical institutions qualified to perform liver transplants in Tibet as of the publication of this report.

In 2020, 12 medical institutions performed more than 150 liver transplants. The total number of liver transplants performed in these hospitals accounted for 52.6% of all cases in China (Table 3-1).

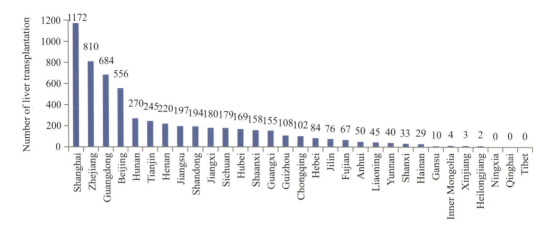

▲ Figure 3-3 Distribution of liver transplantation cases by provinces (autonomous regions and cities) in China in 2020 (not including Hong Kong, Macao, and Taiwan regions)

Table 3-1 Top 12 medical institutions to perform liver transplantation cases in 2020 (not including Hong Kong, Macao, and Taiwan regions)		
Region	**Hospital**	**No. Cases**
Shanghai	Renji Hospital Shanghai Jiaotong University School of Medicine	631
Zhejiang	The First Affiliated Hospital, Zhejiang University School of Medicine	432
Shanghai	Fudan University Zhongshan Hospital	256
Zhejiang	Shulan (Hangzhou) Hospital	255
Tianjin	Tianjin First Central Hospital	245
Shanghai	Huashan Hospital Affiliated to Fudan University	228
Guangdong	The Third Affiliated Hospital,Sun Yat-Sen University	218
Beijing	Beijing Youan Hospital, Capital Medical University	171
Guangdong	The First Affiliated Hospital,Sun Yat-Sen University	163
Henan	First Affiliated Hospital of Zhengzhou	161
Beijing	Beijing Tsinghua Changguang Hospital	160
Shaanxi	The First Affiliated Hospital of Medical College of Xi'an Jiaotong University	154

3.2 Characteristics of liver transplant recipients

In 2020, the mean age of liver transplant recipients in China was 41.0, and their median age was 48.1. Mean BMI (Body Mass Index) of liver transplant recipients was 22.1 kg/m^2 and median BMI was 22.2 kg/m^2. The majority of the recipients were male (74.6%). The major blood types of the recipients were O, A and AB, each accounting for around 30%. Only 10.4% of the recipients had AB blood type (Table 3–2). The average age of pediatric liver transplant recipients was 2.6 years old. There were 689 liver transplant recipients under 1 year old (11.8%), and 333 cases (5.7%) from 1 to 7 years old (not including 7 years old). There were 95 cases (1.6%) from 7 to 12 years old (not including 12 years old), and 62 cases (1.1%) from 12 to 18 years old.

Table 3–2 Characteristics of liver transplant recipients in China in 2020 (not including Hong Kong, Macao, and Taiwan regions)		
Variable	Mean±SD	Proportion（%）
Age	41.0±21.5	—
BMI（kg/m^2）	22.1±4.5	—
Gender		
Male	—	74.6
Female	—	25.4
Type of blood		
Type O	—	30.8
Type A	—	29.7
Type B	—	29.1
Type AB	—	10.4

3.3 Quality analysis of liver transplantation

3.3.1 Major clinical indicators of liver transplantation

In 2020, the mean cold ischemia time, mean length of anhepatic phase, mean intraoperative blood loss, and mean volume of red blood cell (RBC) transfusion of LDLT in China were lower than those of DDLT. Average length of operation of LDLT was slightly higher than that of DDLT (Figure 3–4, Figure 3–5, Figure 3–6, Figure 3–7, Figure 3–8).

3.3.2 Pre- and post-operative variation of total serum bilirubin

In 2020, we analyzed the pre- and post-operative variation of total serum bilirubin in DDLT recipients and LDLT recipients. There was a significant decline in the mean score of post-operative total serum bilirubin in recipients (Table 3–3).

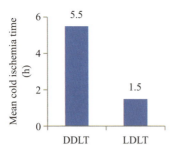

▲ **Figure 3-4** The average cold ischemic time of liver transplantation in 2020 (not including Hong Kong, Macao, and Taiwan regions)

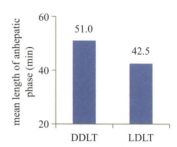

▲ **Figure 3-5** The mean length of anhepatic phase of liver transplantation in 2020 (not including Hong Kong, Macao, and Taiwan regions)

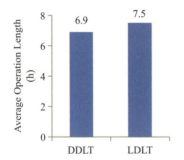

▲ **Figure 3-6** Average operation length for liver transplantation in 2020(not including Hong Kong, Macao, and Taiwan regions)

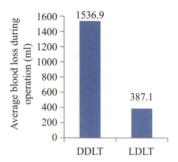

▲ **Figure 3-7** Average blood loss during liver transplantation in 2020(not including Hong Kong, Macao, and Taiwan regions)

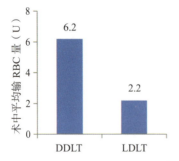

▲ **Figure 3-8** The average amount of RBC transfused during liver transplantation in 2020 (not including Hong Kong, Macao, and Taiwan regions)

3.3.3 Post-operative clinical situation of liver transplant recipients

3.3.3.1 30-day post-operative complications

In 2020, the occurrence rate of 30-day post-operative complications of DDLT recipients was 32.7%. Pleural effusion (20.6%), post-operative infection (13.8%) and intra-abdominal/abscesses (12.6%) were the major complications. The occurrence rate of 30-day post-operative complications of LDLT recipients was 19.4%. Post-operative infection (8.6%), pleural effusion (5.4%) and vascular complications (5.3%) were the major types.

Table 3–3   The average value of total serum bilirubin pre- and post- liver transplantation in 2020 (not including Hong Kong, Macao, and Taiwan regions)

Time	Average value of total serum bilirubin (μmol/L)	
	DDLT	LDLT
Preoperation	242.4	223.0
1 week after operation	65.0	47.2
2 weeks after operation	46.9	26.5
1 month after operation	31.8	16.6
3 months after operation	19.3	9.9
6 months after operation	20.0	10.8

3.3.3.2 30-day post-operative mortality rate

In 2020, the 30–day mortality rate of DDLT recipients was 5.7%, the 30–day mortality rate of LDLT recipients was 3.4%.

3.3.3.3 Survival rate of liver transplant recipients and transplant grafts

We analyzed the data from 2015 to 2020 to see the survival rate of liver transplant recipients and transplant grafts. The results are shown below:

Cumulative survival rate of DDLT recipients in China was 83.6% at 1 year, and 74.9% at 3 years. Cumulative survival rate of LDLT recipients was 91.8% at 1 year, and 88.7% at 3 years.

Cumulative graft survival rate of DDLT in China was 82.9% at 1 year and 73.8% at 3 years; while cumulative graft survival rate of LDLT was 91.1% at 1 year and 87.6% at 3 years (Table 3–4).

Table 3–4   Survival rate of liver transplant recipients/transplant 2015–2020 (not including Hong Kong, Macao, and Taiwan regions)

Group	1–year survival rate after operation (%)		3–year survival rate after operation (%)	
	Recipient	Graft	Recipient	Graft
DDLT	83.6	82.9	74.9	73.8
LDLT	91.8	91.1	88.7	87.6

3.3.3.4 Tumor-free survival after liver transplantation of hepatocellular carcinoma patients

From 2015 to 2020, the tumor-free survival after liver transplantation of hepatocellular carcinoma patients was 77.2% at 1 year, and 63.1% at 3 years.

3.4 Features and Prospects

3.4.1 Pediatric liver transplantation has been developing rapidly

In 2020, 1179 pediatric liver transplants were performed in China, accounting for 20.2% of the total number of transplants, a 7.7% increase compared to the 1095 cases performed in 2019. Among them, 816 cases were from living donors. Of the 363 cases of DDLT in children, whole liver transplantation accounted for 42.7%, reduced sized liver transplantation accounted for 3.0%, and split liver transplantation accounted for 54.3%. The most common indication for liver transplantation in children in China was biliary atresia (72.3%).

3.4.2 Living-related Donor Liver Transplantation (LDLT) accounts for a large proportion

In 2020, LDLT made up for 15.2% (888 cases) of total. At the meantime, among all pediatric liver transplants, LDLT accounted for 69.2%. This number reflected the close relationship among family members in China. In children's LDLT in China, the top three types of liver transplantation are the left lateral lobe (78.2%), the enlarged left lateral lobe (8.6%), and the left lobe (excluding the middle hepatic vein, 5.0%).

3.4.3 Liver transplantation after hepatic carcinoma accounts for a large proportion

As a country with high incidence of hepatic carcinoma, China saw 41.5% of DDLT recipients with malignant tumor in 2020. Hangzhou Criteria for Liver Transplantation in hepatocellular carcinoma was recognized by the academic community and had wide clinical application. Evidence showed that the Criteria have given more HCC patients access to liver transplantation and furthermore, it keeps the survival rate of the recipients at the same level with the international standards.

3.4.4 Exploring innovative surgery and liver transplant techniques

Several transplant centers implemented liver transplantation vascular anastomosis technology, where the anastomosis site has been changed from gastroduodenal artery to splenic artery, significantly improving postoperative liver blood flow and reduced the incidence of biliary complications. Physicians have carried out non-ischemic liver transplants, and have implemented the paired donor exchange supported domino liver transplants, i.e., performing liver exchange between two patients both with metabolic liver disease, thus realized organ transplantation without donation, etc.

3.4.5 Standards and regulations for quality management and control have been established and implemented

We have improved the donor liver quality maintenance and quality assessment system, to enhance the quality of donor liver, reduce the complication rates, as well as advance the recipients survival rates. We have strengthened the monitoring of important post-operative complications, including early graft dysfunction, acute kidney injury and new-onset diabetes, etc. With more scientific and precise quality control systems, we have achieved a significant improvement in clinical service quality and efficacy of liver transplantation across the country.

3.4.6 Scientific monitoring the liver transplant data and valuable information mining

We have strengthened the construction of information system, conducted clinical research based on big data and precise management, promoted the use of evidence-based medicine to guide clinical decision-making. We have been gathering clinical resources to conduct high-quality multi-center clinical research on liver transplantation, and have been dedicated to promoting the clinical translation and application of research findings, thus promote the development of liver transplantation.

3.4.7 Challenges brought by the COVID-19 pandemic

Quantity and quality of liver transplantation in China has been improved steadily in recent years, making China one of the top players in the world. At the beginning of 2020, due to the impact of the COVID-19 pandemic, the number of liver transplants nationwide from January to May decreased compared with the same period in 2019. Nonetheless, since June, the number had exceeded the level of the same period in 2019. According to incomplete statistics, 3 liver transplant recipients were diagnosed with COVID-19 after transplantation, which brought tough challenge to transplant centers. These 3 recipients had been transferred to designated hospitals for treatment, after which their nucleic acid tests of COVID-19 throat swabs all turned negative.

3.4.8 Prospect of split liver transplantation (SLT)

In 2020, among all DDLT, there were 387 cases of SLT. The implementation of SLT can effectively expand the source of donor liver and reduce the waiting time of patients for transplantation. It could especially help tackle the issue of organ shortage for pediatric recipients: more than 50% of the recipients of the above mentioned 387 cases were pediatric patients. In split liver transplantation in China, the top three types of liver transplantation are the left lateral lobe (26.9%), the right lobe + segment Ⅳ (22.0%), and the right lobe (including the middle hepatic vein, 19.1%). The selection criteria for livers suitable for splitting and recipients who can receive SLT need to be further clarified in order to achieve more optimal allocation of livers.

Chapter 4 Kidney Transplantation in China

The data showed in this chapter are mainly based on data analysis from the Chinese Scientific Registry of Kidney Transplantation (CSRKT). The statistics represent that of the Mainland China, not including Hong Kong, Macao, and Taiwan.

CSRKT is an official online registration system of kidney transplantation established by the National Health Commission of China. It requires national medical institutions qualified for kidney transplantation to report relevant information in a timely and complete manner. CSRKT, the only system in China for the registration of kidney recipients, provides each transplantation center with a scientific management tool based on the dynamic and scientific analysis of kidney transplants in Mainland China, which sets the scientific foundation for the national regulatory authorities to formulate transplant-related policies and regulations. Thus far, CSRKT has become the key information system of China organ transplantation and one of the academic exchange platforms for kidney transplantation.

4.1 Distribution of medical institutions qualified for kidney transplantation

By December 31st, 2020, there were 132 medical institutions qualified for kidney transplantation in China. The top 10 provinces (autonomous regions and cities) with the greatest number of qualified institutions were Guangdong (18), Beijing (13), Shandong (10), Hunan (9), Zhejiang (8), Shanghai (7), Guangxi (6), Henan (6), Hubei (6), and Liaoning (5) (Figure 4–1).

From 2015 to 2020, 63 042 cases of kidney transplantation had been performed in China, including 52 285 cases of DD (Deceased Donor) kidney transplantation and 10 757 from living donors. There were 11 037 cases performed in 2020, with a 9.0% decline compared with that in 2019. Specifically, there were 9399 cases of DD kidney transplantation, which was 9.5% lower compared with that in 2019; and 1638 cases of living-related transplants, a 5.6% decline compared with that in 2019 (Figure 4–2).

In 2020, 149 kidney-related multi-organ transplantations were performed across the country, decreasing by 33.5% compared with 2019 (Figure 4–3). Among these transplantations, 39 cases were liver-kidney transplantation; 103 cases were pancreas-kidney transplantation; and 7 cases were heart-kidney transplantation.

In 2020, the top 10 provinces (autonomous regions and cities) with the most kidney-related multi-organ transplantation performed were Guangdong, Shandong, Guangxi, Tianjin, Beijing, Shanghai, Zhejiang, Hainan, Henan, Hunan, and Jiangsu (Figure 4–4). The medical institutions with the greatest number of kidney-related multi-organ transplantation performed in 2020 were The Second Affiliated Hospital of Guangzhou Medical University (59), The Affiliated Hospital of Qingdao University (16), The Second Affiliated Hospital of Guangxi Medical University (13), The First Affiliated Hospital, Sun Yat-Sen University (10), Tianjin First Central Hospital (8), The First Affiliated Hospital Zhejiang

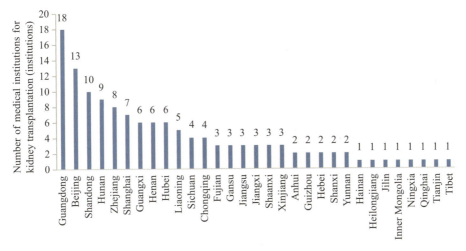

▲ **Figure 4−1 Distribution of medical institution qualified for kidney transplantation in China (By the end of 2020, not including Hong Kong, Macao, and Taiwan regions)**

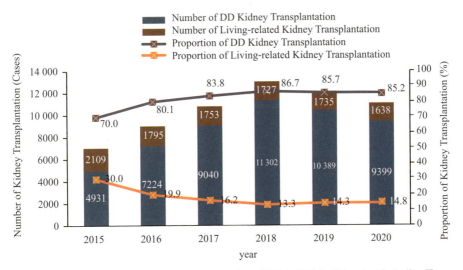

▲ **Figure 4−2 Kidney transplantation cases from 2015 to 2020 in China (not including Hong Kong, Macao and Taiwan regions)**

University School of Medicine (4), Beijing Tsinghua Changgung Hospital Affiliated to Tsinghua University (3), Fudan University Zhongshan Hospital (3), The Second Affiliated Hospital of Hainan Medical University (3), People's Hospital of Henan University of Chinese Medicine (People's Hospital of Zhengzhou)(3), and The Third Affiliated Hospital, Sun Yat-Sen University (3) (Table 4–1).

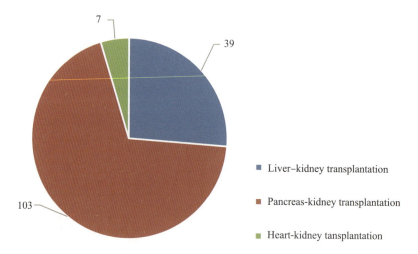

■ Liver–kidney transplantation

■ Pancreas-kidney transplantation

■ Heart-kidney tansplantation

▲ **Figure 4–3** **Kidney-related multi-organ transplantations in China in 2020 (not including Hong Kong, Macao, and Taiwan regions)**

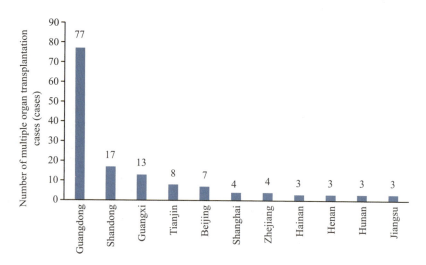

▲ **Figure 4–4** **Top 10 provinces (autonomous regions and cities) of kidney-related multi-organ transplantation in 2020 (not including Hong Kong, Macao, and Taiwan regions)**

Table 4-1	Top 10 medical institutions to perform kidney-related multi-organ transplantation in 2020 (not including Hong Kong, Macao, and Taiwan regions)	
Region	**Hospital**	**No. Cases**
Guangdong	The Second Affiliated Hospital of Guangzhou Medical University	59
Shandong	The Affiliated Hospital of Qingdao University	16
Guangxi	The Second Affiliated Hospital of Guangxi Medical University	13
Guangdong	The First Affiliated Hospital, Sun Yat-Sen University	10
Tianjin	Tianjin First Central Hospital	8
Zhejiang	The First Affiliated Hospital Zhejiang University School of Medicine	4
Beijing	Beijing Tsinghua Changgung Hospital Affiliated to Tsinghua University	3
Shanghai	Fudan University Zhongshan Hospital	3
Hainan	The Second Affiliated Hospital of Hainan Medical University	3
Henan	People's Hospital of Henan University of Chinese Medicine (People's Hospital of Zhengzhou)	3
Guangdong	The Third Affiliated Hospital, Sun Yat-Sen University	3

Transplantation for children ($<$18 years) has drawn more attention in recent years. In 2020, the number of pediatric kidney transplants accounted for 2.7% of the gross domestic cases of kidney transplants in China (Figure 4-5).

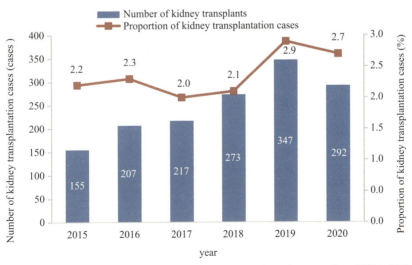

▲ **Figure 4-5** **Number and proportion of kidney transplantation cases from 2015 to 2020 (not including Hong Kong, Macao, and Taiwan regions)**

In 2020, the top 10 provinces to perform kidney-related multi-organ transplantation were Guangdong, Zhejiang, Shandong, Hunan, Henan, Shanghai, Beijing, Hubei, Sichuan, and Guangxi (Figure 4–6).

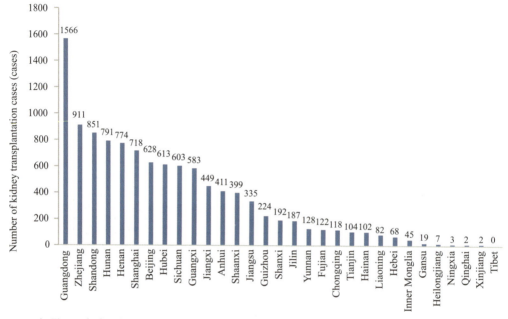

▲ **Figure 4–6** **Distribution of kidney transplantation by provinces (autonomous regions and cities) in 2020 (not including Hong Kong, Macao, and Taiwan regions)**

10 medical institutions had performed more than 250 cases of kidney transplantation, accounting for 32.6% of all cases in 2020. 5 medical institutions had performed 200~249 cases; 25 medical institutions had performed 100~199 cases; 22 medical institutions had performed 50~99 cases. 34 medical institutions had been performed 10~49 cases; and 18 medical institutions had performed 1~9 cases. Additionally, 18 medical institutions had not performed kidney transplantation (7 of which had not performed kidney transplantation from 2018 to 2020). Table 4–2 shows the number and proportion of kidney transplantation cases in 2020.

No. Cases	Number of medical institutions	Proportion (%)
Table 4–2 Distribution of kidney transplantation by number of cases performed in 2020 (not including Hong Kong, Macao, and Taiwan regions)		
≥ 250	10	32.6
200~249	5	9.9
100~199	25	31.6

(Continuations)

No. Cases	Number of medical institutions	Proportion (%)
50～99	22	15.4
10～49	34	9.7
1～9	18	0.8
0	18	0

A pattern of regional advantages has become apparent in 2020. 9 provinces (autonomous regions and cities) have performed more than 600 cases of kidney transplantation, accounting for 67.5% of all cases in 2020 (Table 4–3).

Table 4–3 Distribution of provincial kidney transplantation by number of cases performed in 2020 (not including Hong Kong, Macao, and Taiwan regions)

No. Cases	Number of provinces (autonomous regions and cities)	Proportion (%)
≥ 600	9	67.5
400～599	3	13.1
200～399	3	8.7
100～199	7	8.6
1～99	8	2.1
0	1	0.0

In 2020, the top 10 provinces (autonomous regions and cities) with the greatest number of DD kidney transplantations were Guangdong, Shandong, Hunan, Zhejiang, Shanghai, Henan, Beijing, Guangxi, Hubei and Jiangxi, accounting for 75.3% of the total number of DD cases in China in 2020 (Figure 4–7). The top 10 medical institutions to perform DD kidney transplantation were Renji Hospital Shanghai Jiaotong University School of Medicine (412), The first Affiliated Hospital of Xian Jiaotong University (365), The First Affiliated Hospital, Sun Yat-Sen University (344), The Second Affiliated Hospital of Guangzhou Medical University (290), The Second Affiliated Hospital of Guangxi Medical University (288), Shulan (Hangzhou) Hospital (279), The First Affiliated Hospital, Zhejiang University School of Medicine (257), The First Affiliated Hospital of Zhengzhou University (239), The Affiliated Hospital of Qingdao University (223), West China Hospital, Sichuan University (222). (Table 4–4).

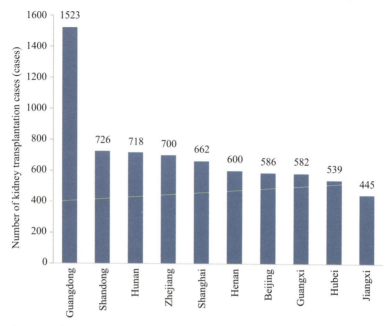

▲ Figure 4–7 **Top 10 provinces (autonomous regions and cities) to perform DD kidney transplantation (not including Hong Kong, Macao, and Taiwan regions)**

Region	Hospital	No. Cases
Table 4–4 **Top ten medical institutions to perform DD kidney transplantation cases in 2020 (not including Hong Kong, Macao, and Taiwan regions)**		
Shanghai	Renji Hospital Shanghai Jiaotong University School of Medicine	412
Shaanxi	The first Affiliated Hospital of Xian Jiaotong University	365
Guangdong	The First Affiliated Hospital, Sun Yat-Sen University	344
Guangdong	The Second Affiliated Hospital of Guangzhou Medical University	290
Guangxi	The Second Affiliated Hospital of Guangxi Medical University	288
Zhejiang	Shulan (Hangzhou) Hospital	279
Zhejiang	The First Affiliated Hospital, Zhejiang University School of Medicine	257
Henan	The First Affiliated Hospital of Zhengzhou University	239
Shandong	The Affiliated Hospital of Qingdao University	223
Sichuan	West China Hospital, Sichuan University	222

The top 10 provinces (autonomous regions and cities) to perform living-related kidney transplantations were Sichuan, Anhui, Zhejiang, Henan, Shandong, Hubei, Hunan, Shanghai, Guangdong, and Beijing (Figure 4–8). The top 10 medical institutions to perform living-related kidney transplantation were West China Hospital, Sichuan University (269), The First Affiliated Hospital of USTC (233), The First Affiliated Hospital, Zhejiang University School of Medicine (201), The First Affiliated Hospital of Zhengzhou University (93), The First Affiliated Hospital of Anhui Medical University (64), Henan Provincial People's Hospital (54), The Second Xiangya Hospital of Central South University (53), Tongji Hospital, Tongji Medical College of HUST (49), the First Affiliated Hospital of Shandong First Medical University (Shandong Provincial Qianfoshan Hospital) (41), Sichuan Provincial People's Hospital (40) (Table 4–5).

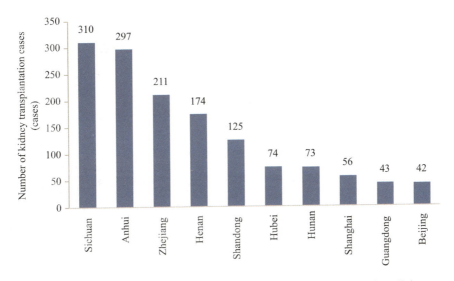

▲ **Figure 4–8** **Top 10 provinces (autonomous regions and cities) to perform living-related kidney transplantation (not including Hong Kong, Macao, and Taiwan regions)**

Region	Hospital	No. Cases
Sichuan	West China Hospital, Sichuan University	269
Anhui	The First Affiliated Hospital of USTC	233
Zhejiang	The First Affiliated Hospital, Zhejiang University School of Medicine	201
Henan	The First Affiliated Hospital of Zhengzhou University	93

Table 4–5 Top 10 medical institution to perform living-related kidney transplantation (not including Hong Kong, Macao, and Taiwan regions)

(Continuations)

Region	Hospital	No. Cases
Anhui	The First Affiliated Hospital of Anhui Medical University	64
Henan	Henan Provincial People's Hospital	54
Hunan	The Second Xiangya Hospital of Central South University	53
Hubei	Tongji Hospital, Tongji Medical College of HUST	49
Shandong	the First Affiliated Hospital of Shandong First Medical University (Shandong Provincial Qianfoshan Hospital)	41
Sichuan	Sichuan Provincial People's Hospital	40

4.2 Geographic characteristics of kidney transplantation recipients

According to the data analysis of kidney transplantation in Mainland China, the mean age of the recipients was (40.2 ± 12.0). Mean BMI (Body Mass Index) of the recipients was (22.0±3.4) kg/m^2. The median duration of pretransplant dialysis was 482 days. The majority of the recipients were male (69.3%). Only 9.7% of the recipients had AB blood type (Table 4–6).

Table 4–6 Data of kidney transplantation recipients (not including Hong Kong, Macao, and Taiwan regions)		
Variable		**Mean ± SD**
Recipient age (years)		40.2±12.0
BMI（kg/m^2）		22.0±3.4
Dialysis duration		**Median (IQR)**
Preoperative dialysis duration (days)		482 (244~1028)
Recipient blood type		**Proportion (%)**
O	3695	33.5
A	3193	28.9
B	3083	27.9
AB	1066	9.7
Gender		**Proportion (%)**
Male	7652	69.3
Female	3385	30.7

Note: IQR, Interquartile range

Among all recipients: Pediatric kidney transplant recipients ($<$ 18 years) accounted for 292 cases (2.7%); recipients aged 18–30 years accounted for 1792 cases (16.2%); recipients aged 30–50 years accounted for 6259 cases (56.7%); recipients aged 50–65 years accounted for 2520 cases (22.8%); transplantations among the elderly ($\geqslant$ 65 years) accounted for 174 cases (1.6%).

4.3 Quality and safety analysis of kidney transplantation

4.3.1 Ischemia time of donor kidney for DD kidney transplantation

The analysis of living-related and DD kidney transplantation cases in 2020 showed that the average cold ischemia time of the donor kidney did not exceed 6 hours (Table 4–7). 99.9% of living donor kidney transplants between relatives and 99.7% of DD kidney transplants have a cold ischemia time of less than or equal to 24 hours; 98.4% of living donor kidney transplants between relatives and 83.8% of DD kidney transplants have a warm ischemic time of less than or equal to 10 minutes (Table 4–8).

Table 4–7 Ischemia time of donor kidney in 2020 (not including Hong Kong, Macao, and Taiwan regions)

Variable	Living donor (Mean $\pm$ SD)	DD (Mean $\pm$ SD)
Kidney cold ischemia time (hour)	1.9±1.2	5.8±3.9
Kidney warm ischemia time (minute)	3.1±2.3	6.4±5.1

Table 4–8 Proportion of ischemia time of donor kidney in 2020 (not including Hong Kong, Macao, and Taiwan regions)

Variable	Living donor (%)	DD (%)
Kidney cold ischemia time $\leqslant$ 24 (hour)	99.9	99.7
Kidney warm ischemia time $\leqslant$ 10 (minute)	98.4	83.8

4.3.2 Changes of the pre- and post-transplant recipient's serum creatinine value

In 2020, 11 037 cases of kidney transplantation were performed in China. According to the CSRKT, serum creatinine values were analyzed in 4 follow-up periods (pre-operation, 30 days, 180 days, and 360 days after surgery) of living donor and DD donor. (Table 4–9).

Table 4–9 Mean value of recipient's serum creatinine before and after kidney transplantation in China in 2020 (not including Hong Kong, Macao, and Taiwan regions)

Time	Living donor (μmol/L)	DD (μmol/L)
Before surgery	1012.0	932.5

(Continuations)

Time	Living donor (μmol/L)	DD (μmol/L)
30 days after surgery	119.2	145.7
180 days after surgery	116.2	122.9
360 days after surgery	117.3	115.7

4.3.3 Overview of adverse event after kidney transplantation

Adverse events after kidney transplantation usually include: delayed function of allograft, acute rejection, death of recipient and renal allograft loss. According to the retrospective analysis of cases in 2020, the major adverse events are presented in Table 4–10 and Table 4–11. The 30–day postoperative mortality rate was 0.3%. No major complication occurred among cases involving living donors.

Table 4–10 Rate of adverse events after kidney transplantation in 2020 (not including Hong Kong, Macao, and Taiwan regions)

Adverse event	Living donor (%)	DD (%)
Delayed graft function	2.4	12.2
Acute rejection	1.8	4.8
Infection	1.1	2.5
Recipient death	0.7	1.7
All-cause graft loss	1.0	3.6

Table 4–11 Rate of overall adverse events after kidney transplantation in 2020 (not including Hong Kong, Macao, and Taiwan regions)

Adverse event	Overall adverse event (%)
Delayed graft function	8.7
Acute rejection	9.7
Infection	6.8
Recipient death	12.6
All-cause graft loss	12.6

4.3.4 Survival analysis of kidney transplant recipient and graft

From 2015 to 2020, there were 63 042 cases of kidney transplantation performed in China. Results of the survival analysis of transplantation recipients and grafts are shown below:

- 1–year survival rate after transplantation: The 1–year human/kidney survival rate of living-related kidney transplantation between relatives is 99.3%/98.7%; the 1-year human/kidney survival rate of DD kidney transplantation is 97.8%/95.8%. (Table 4-12).

- 3-year survival rate after transplantation: 3-year survival rate/kidney survival rate for living-related kidney transplantation among relatives is 98.8%/96.8%; 3-year survival rate/kidney survival rate for DD kidney transplantation is 96.8%/93.2% (Table 4-12).

Table 4-12 Survival rate of kidney transplantation after surgery (not including Hong Kong, Macao, and Taiwan regions)

Donor type	1 year after surgery		3 years after surgery	
	Recipient (%)	Allograft (%)	Recipient (%)	Allograft (%)
Living donor	99.3	98.7	98.8	96.8
Deceased Donor	97.8	95.8	96.8	93.2

4.4 Features and prospects

4.4.1 DD kidney transplantation as the dominating type

Chinese kidney transplantation has entered a bright new stage of benign development. In the past 5 years, the number of DD kidney transplantation cases accounted for more than 80% of all cases, and it was 85.2% in 2020. Provinces including Guangdong, Shandong, Hunan, Zhejiang, Shanghai, etc., are with obvious regional advantages. Kidney transplants for children are mainly carried out in provinces including Guangdong, Henan, Shanghai, etc. Application and promotion of pediatric kidney donation are worthy of notice.

The principle of regional allocation of organs and the establishment of green channels for organ transport have shortened the cold ischemic time of donor kidneys for DD kidney transplantation. The 1-year and 3-year survival rates of living-related kidney transplantation and DD kidney transplantation were satisfactory. In 2020, there were 149 cases of kidney-related multi-organ transplantation, of which 69.1% were pancreas-kidney transplantation, which were mainly carried out in Guangdong, Shandong, Guangxi, Tianjin and Beijing.

4.4.2 Continuous promotion of Chinese kidney transplantation quality improvement program

Kidney transplantation quality control center has always sought to build a platform which promote the development of kidney transplantation in China. Its goal is to play a leading role in the field, strengthen the management of the medical quality of human organ transplantation, realize the continuous improvement of the national kidney transplant medical quality and service, and narrow the medical gap between transplant centers. A series of quality control standards and technical norms have been promulgated and continuously updated in the past two years. The content involves various technical fields of kidney transplantation, which has great clinical guiding significance, so as to realize a virtuous circle from medical quality assessment (control) to medical quality improvement, and continuously promote the development of kidney transplantation in China.

4.4.3 Research hotspots and breakthroughs in kidney transplantation

For a long time in the future, the shortage of organ donor and allograft rejection are still the crucial limiting factors for the development of kidney transplantation. Over the years, domestic researchers have been committed to connecting the research in immunology, stem cell, and genetic engineering with organ transplantation, and carrying out basic and clinical research. It provides a theoretical and practical basis for further optimizing the medical quality of kidney transplantation. Breakthroughs have been made in research hotspots such as ischemia-reperfusion injury, acute rejection, chronic graft failure, renal fibrosis, maintenance and utilization of marginal donor kidneys, transplant-related viral infections, clinical indicator monitoring and early warning after kidney transplantation, adult kidney transplantation with double-kidney from low-weight infant donor, etc.

Chapter 5 Heart Transplantation in China

The data showed in this chapter are mainly based on data analysis from the China Heart Transplant Registry (CHTR), not including Hongkong, Macao, and Taiwan, China.

CHTR is the official registry system established by the National Health Committee of China. All transplant centers qualified for liver transplantation are required to submit transplantation data in a timely and complete manner. The data of CHTR include characteristics of recipients and donors, situation of transplant surgeries, immunosuppressant, in-hospital and long-term outcomes. CHTR releases regular reports regarding the national, regional, and center-specific heart transplantation volumes, results of data audit, and patient outcomes via comprehensive analysis of collected data. Based on those analyses and reports, CHTR summaries results and experience on donor heart procurement and preservation, donor-recipients matching, and clinical transplantation management. Furthermore, CHTR provides vital information for the constitution of relative regulations, laws and guidelines for the national administrative authorities.

5.1 Distribution of medical institutions qualified for heart transplantation

By December 31st, 2020, a total of 56 medical institutions in China were qualified for heart transplantation. The top ten provinces (autonomous regions and cities) with the largest number of heart transplant hospitals are Guangdong (6), Zhejiang (6), Beijing (5), Hubei (5), Henan (3), Tianjin (3), Yunnan (3), Fujian (2), Guangxi (2), Liaoning (2), Shandong (2), Shanghai (2) and Sichuan (2). There was no heart transplant hospital in Tibet, Gansu, Guizhou, Jiangxi, and Jilin as of the publication of this report (Figure 5–1).

From 2015 to 2020, a total of 2819 heart transplantation cases were reported in China (Figure 5–2). In 2020, a total of 38 heart transplantation centers performed 557 cases of heart transplantation, including 52 pediatric transplantation and 7 cases of heart-lung transplantation. The number of transplants decreased by 18.0% compared with 2019. The distribution of the number of heart transplants by provinces is shown in Figure 5–3. In 2020, except for Hong Kong, Macao, and Taiwan, the top 10 hospitals ranked by the total number of transplantation cases were Fuwai Hospital, Chinese Academy of Medical Sciences (78), Union Hospital of Huazhong University of Science and Technology (73), Guangdong Provincial People's Hospital (54), People's Hospital of Zhengzhou

(44), Zhongshan Hospital Affiliated to Fudan University (43), The First Affiliated Hospital, Zhejiang University School of Medicine (26), Fujian Medical University Union Hospital (25), Nanjing First Hospital (22), Sun Yat-sen Memorial Hospital, Sun Yat-sen University (18), and Wuhan Asia Heart Hospital (16) (Figure 5–4).

5.2 Characteristics of heart transplant recipients

In 2020, the median age of heart transplant recipients was 50.0 years old. The majority of the recipients were male (74.7%). The median BMI (Body Mass Index) of recipients was 22.2kg/m^2.

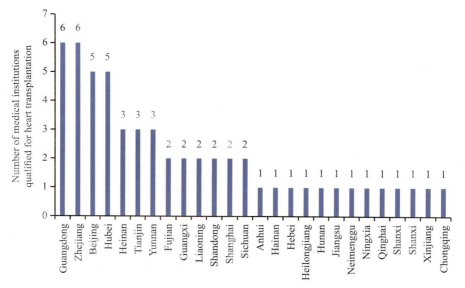

▲ **Figure 5–1** **Distribution of hospitals qualified for heart transplantation in China in 2020 (not including Hong Kong, Macao, and Taiwan regions)**

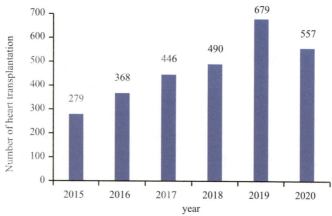

▲ **Figure 5–2** **Number of heart transplantation cases in China from 2015 to 2020 (not including Hong Kong, Macao, and Taiwan regions)**

As for the blood types of transplant recipients, type O accounted for 30.8%, type A accounted for 30.5%, type B accounted for 28.3%, and type AB accounted for 10.4% of all recipients. The median age of adult transplant recipients is 52.0 years, of which 76.1% were males. The median age of child transplant recipients is 10.5 years, of which 56.6% were males (Table 5–1). The main causes of recipients demanding heart transplant were non-ischemic cardiomyopathy and coronary heart disease, accounting for 74.4% and 15.5%, respectively, followed by valvular heart disease (4.4%) and congenital heart disease (3.0%). The main causes of adult recipients were non-ischemic cardiomyopathy (73.3%) and coronary heart disease (16.9%); the main causes of child recipients are non-ischemic cardiomyopathy (84.9%) and congenital heart disease (11.3%).

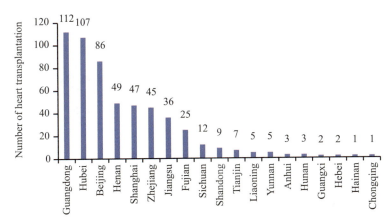

▲ **Figure 5–3** **Distribution of heart transplantation cases in China by provinces (autonomous regions and cities) in 2020 (not including Hong Kong, Macao, and Taiwan regions)**

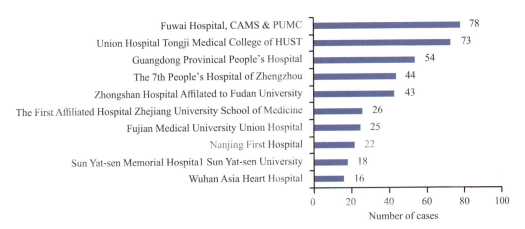

▲ **Figure 5–4** **The top ten hospitals in China by number of heart transplant cases in 2020 (not including Hong Kong, Macao, and Taiwan regions)**

Table 5-1 Characteristics of heart transplant recipients in China in 2020(not including Hong Kong, Macao, and Taiwan regions)			
Variable	**Total** (*N*=557)	**Adult recipient** (*N*=505)	**Pediatric recipient** (*N*=52)
Median age，IQR（year）	50.0 (34.0～59.0)	52.0 (40.0～59.0)	10.5 (3.5～12.5)
Male（%）	74.7	76.1	56.6
Median weight，IQR（kg）	62.3 (54.0～70.0)	54.3 (56.0～71.7)	26.0 (16.0～40.0)
Median height，IQR（cm）	169.0 (161.0～172.0)	170.0 (163.0～173.0)	140.0 (110.0～160.0)
Median BMI，IQR（kg/m^2）	22.2 (19.6～24.6)	22.5 (20.4～24.8)	14.9 (13.0～18.0)
Cause of heart transplantation（%）			
Non-ischemic cardiomyopathy	74.4	73.3	84.9
Coronary Heart Disease	15.5	16.9	1.9
Congenital heart disease	3.0	2.0	11.3
Valvular heart disease	4.4	4.9	0
Others	2.7	2.9	1.9

NOTE: IQR, interquartile range.

5.3　Quality analysis of heart transplantation

5.3.1　Ischemia time

Figure 5-5 shows the distribution of ischemic time of heart transplantation nationwide in 2020. The median ischemic time of heart transplantation in China was 3.7 hours, which decreased compared to the median ischemic time of 4.0 hours in 2019. 83.4% of heart transplant recipients had ischemia time less than or equal to 6 hours, slightly lower than the proportion (84.4%) in 2019.

5.3.2　Application rate of intraoperative and postoperative mechanical circulation support

Figure 5-6 shows the use of intraoperative and postoperative mechanical circulation support of heart transplantation nationwide in 2020. The application rate of intra-aortic balloon pump (IABP) was 19.0%; the application rate of Extracorporeal Membrane Oxygenation (ECMO) was 12.7%; and the application rate of continuous renal replacement therapy (CRRT) was 21.2%, which was higher than the corresponding rates (18.0%, 10.0% and 16.4%, respectively) in 2019.

5.3.3　Postoperative mechanical ventilation time

The median time of mechanical ventilation after heart transplantation in China was 36 hours in 2020 (Figure 5-7), which is greater than the median ischemic time of 27 hours in 2019. 71.5% recipients had mechanical ventilation time less than or equal to 48 hours in 2019, and the proportion was 63.7% in 2020.

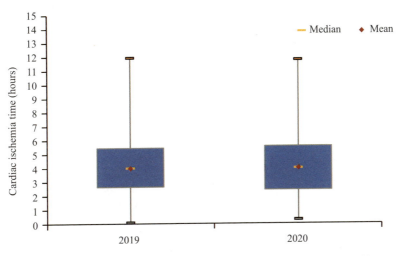

▲ **Figure 5−5   Ischemic time of heart transplantation in China in 2019 and 2020 (not including Hong Kong, Macao, and Taiwan regions)**

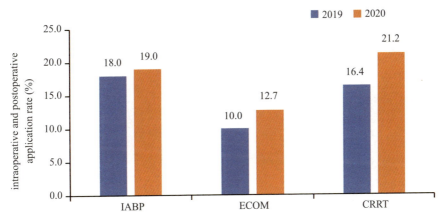

▲ **Figure 5−6   Application of mechanical assistance during and after heart transplantation in China in 2019 and 2020 (not including Hong Kong, Macao, and Taiwan regions）**

5.3.4 In-hospital survival

In 2020, the in-hospital survival rate of heart transplant recipients in China was 88.5%. The incidence of postoperative infection among heart transplant recipients was 26.6%, and the other major postoperative complications were cardiac arrest (5.7%), reoperation (5.7%), tracheotomy (6.3%) and reintubation (7.9%). Among the causes of in-hospital death of heart transplant recipients, multiple organ failure and transplanted heart failure accounted for more than 60% of early deaths (Table 5–2).

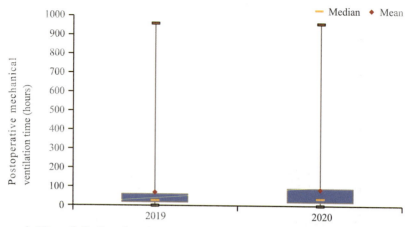

▲ Figure 5−7   Duration of mechanical ventilation after heart transplantation in China in 2019 and 2020 (not including Hong Kong, Macao, and Taiwan regions)

Table 5–2 In-Hospital survival of heart transplant recipients in 2020			
Variable	Proportion（%）		
	Total (*N*=557)	Adult recipient (*N*=505)	Pediatric recipient （*N*=52）
In-hospital survival	88.5	88.0	92.3
Postoperative complications			
Postoperative infection	23.4	22.9	28.3
Cardiac arrest	5.7	5.5	7.6
Second thoracotomy	5.7	5.9	3.8
Tracheotomy	6.3	6.7	1.9
Secondary intubation	7.9	8.4	3.8
Cause of death			
Multiple organ failure	34.4	34.5	33
Transplant heart failure	15.6	27.6	50
Infection	26.6	12.1	17
Others	23.5	25.8	0

5.3.5 Survival analysis

From 2015 to 2020, the 30–day, 1–year, and 3–year survival rate after heart transplantation were 92.6%, 85.3% and 80.4%, respectively. The corresponding survival rates among adult recipients were 92.5%, 85.3%, and 80.4%, respectively; The corresponding survival rates among child recipients were 94.5%, 91.0% and 84.0%, respectively (Table 5–3).

Table 5–3 Survival rate after heart transplantation, 2015–2020			
	30–day survival (%)	1–year survival (%)	3–year survival (%)
All recipients	92.6	85.3	80.4
Adult recipient	92.5	85.3	80.4
Pediatric recipient	94.5	91.0	84.0

5.4 Features and Prospects

Affected by the COVID-19 pandemic, the number of heart transplants nationwide in 2020 has dropped by 18% compared with 2019, but it was still an increase of 14% compared with that of 2018. Three heart transplant centers – Fuwai Hospital, Union Hospital affiliated to Tongji Medical College of Huazhong University of Science and Technology, and Guangdong Provincial People's Hospital had performed more than 50 heart transplant cases in 2020, and the number of transplant cases in Zhengzhou Seventh People's Hospital and Zhongshan Hospital of Fudan University were also more than 40. These transplant centers have maintained a strong capability of medical service capacity in the context of the fight against the COVID-19 pandemic and provided relatively stable medical accessibility for patients awaiting heart transplant in China. However, the top ten heart transplant centers with the largest number of cases performed were concentrated in the central and eastern regions of China. The differences in development of regional heart transplantation capacity still need to be narrowed.

Thanks to the efficient operation of the COTRS and the unremitting efforts of various transplant medical teams, the proportion of cases with a cardiac ischemic time less than or equal to 6 hours in 2020 maintained close to that in 2019, although still far from the situation in Western countries. It is necessary to further optimize the allocation system of donated hearts and strengthen the efficiency of donor procurement and cooperation in transportation. The median time of mechanical ventilation and the proportion of ventilation less than 48 hours after heart transplantation both got worse than that in 2019, suggesting that the quality of perioperative management of recipients needs to be further improved.

In terms of the outcome of heart transplantation, the in-hospital mortality rate of heart transplantation in China in 2020 is higher than that in 2019. Quality control and improvement in the preoperative evaluation and perioperative management of recipients should be improved to further reduce the in-hospital mortality rate.

In the future, the China Heart Transplant Quality Control Center will continue to improve the China Heart Transplant Registration System, to assist newly qualified hospitals for heart transplantation, and to improve the quality of heart transplantation through a series of quality improvement programs.

Chapter 6 Lung Transplantation in China

This Chapter presents information on lung transplantation activity in Mainland China. Data were obtained from the China Lung Transplant Registry (CLuTR), not including Hongkong, Macao and Taiwan, China.

CLuTR is an official registry system of lung transplantation established by the National Health Commission of China. It collects the pre-operative, mid-operative, post-operative and follow-up data of recipients and essential information of donors. The CluTR has been committed to analyzing the lung transplantation related data in a dynamic and scientific manner, which sets the scientific foundation for the national regulatory authorities to formulate transplant-related policies and regulations.

6.1 Distribution of medical institutions qualified for lung transplantation

By December 31th, 2020, a total of 43 medical institutions in Mainland China, excluding Hongkong, Macao, and Taiwan regions, were qualified for lung transplantation. These institutions were from 21 provinces across the country, and mainly concentrated in East and North China. The top 10 provinces (autonomous regions and cities) with the most medical institutions qualified for lung transplantation were: Beijing (5), Guangdong (5), Hubei(4), Zhejiang(4), Tianjin (3), Shanghai (3), Liaoning (2), Sichuan (2), Henan(2), and Guangxi (2). There was no lung transplant hospital in Hebei, Shanxi, Jilin, Jiangxi, Chongqing, Guizhou, Tibet, Gansu, Qinghai, and Ningxia s of the publication of this report (Figure 6–1).

From January 1st, 2015 to December 31st, 2020, 2026 cases of lung transplantation were reported through CluTR. Over the 6 years, 118 cases, 204 cases, 299 cases, 403 cases, 489 cases, 513 cases have been performed each year (Figure 6–2), showing an upward trend over time.

In 2020, a total of 29 lung transplantation centers performed lung transplants. The 10 centers with most cases performed were Wuxi People's Hospital (156), China-Japan Friendship Hospital (77), The First Affiliated Hospital of Guangzhou Medical University (76), Shanghai Pulmonary Hospital (40), The First Affiliated Hospital of Zhengzhou University (39), The Second Affiliated Hospital, Zhejiang University School of Medicine (26), The First Affiliated Hospital, Zhejiang University School of Medicine (18), Henan Provincial People's Hospital (15), Sichuan Provincial People's Hospital (12), and The First Affiliated Hospital of USTC (Anhui Provincial Hospital) (9) (Figure 6–3).

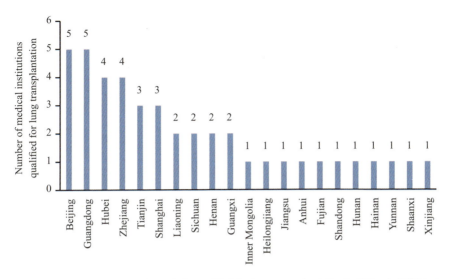

▲ **Figure 6−1** **Distribution of hospitals qualified for lung transplantation in China in 2020 (not including Hong Kong, Macao, and Taiwan regions)**

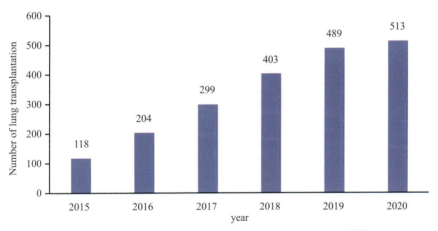

▲ **Figure 6−2** **Number of lung transplantation cases in China from 2015 to 2020 (not including Hong Kong, Macao, and Taiwan regions)**

6.2 Characteristics of lung transplant recipients

In 2020, the median cold ischemia time of single lung transplantation was 6.5 hours (IQR 5.0~7.5); that of double lung transplantation was 8.5 hours (IQR 7.0~9.5). Proportions of single lung transplantation recipients whose cold ischemia time was less than 2 hours, between 2~4 hours, between 4~6 hours, between 6~8 hours and more than 8 hours were 4.8%, 16.3%, 22.3%, 48.2% and 8.4%, respectively. That distribution for double lung transplantation recipients was 0.0%, 3.7%, 15.4%, 23.4% and 57.5% respectively (Figure 6–4).

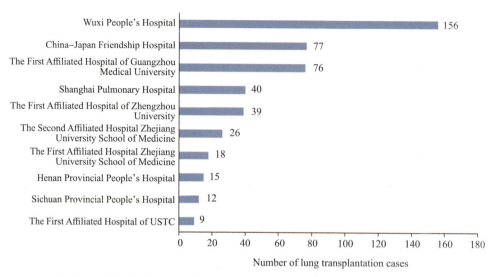

▲ **Figure 6-3** **Top 10 hospitals by number of lung transplant cases in 2020 (not including Hong Kong, Macao, and Taiwan regions)**

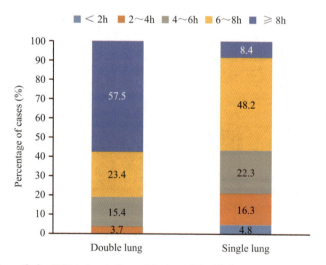

▲ **Figure 6-4** **Cold ischemia time of single and double lung transplant recipients in 2020 (not including Hong Kong, Macao, and Taiwan regions)**

In 2020, among all lung transplant recipients, male accounted for 66.8%. Median age of the recipients was 54.9±12.8. Recipients older than 60 years accounted for nearly half of all recipients (48.0%). The median BMI (Body Mass Index) of recipients was (20.7±3.5) kg/m². As for blood type, type O accounted for 31.3%, type A accounted for 29.2%, type B accounted for 28.7%, and type AB accounted for 9.7% of all recipients. 32.2% of all the recipients had used hormonal drugs, and 13.8% of them were hospitalized in the ICU. As for heart function status, patients with total restriction of daily activities (NYHA IV) accounted for 24.3%; patients with severe symptoms and required hospitalization accounted for 16.1% (Table 6–1).

Variable	Proportion (%)	Variable	Proportion (%)
Gender		Blood type	
Male	66.8	O	31.3
Female	33.2	A	29.2
Age (year)		B	28.7
< 18	1.1	AB	9.7
18—35	8.5	History of hormone use	
36—49	16.1	Ever	32.2
50—59	26.3	Never	67.8
60—64	27.3	Hospitalization before transplantation	
≥ 65	20.7	ICU	13.8
BMI (kg/m^2)		Hospitalization	70.1
< 18.5	27.9	Not hospitalized	14.7
18.6~23.9	51.5	Heart function state before transplantation	
≥ 24.0	17.1	No activity restrictions (NYHA I / II)	1.8
		Partially limited daily activities (NYHA III)	53.4
		Completely restricted daily activities (NYHA IV)	24.3
		Serious illness requiring hospitalization	16.1

Table 6–1　Characteristics of lung transplant recipients in 2020 (not including Hong Kong, Macao, and Taiwan regions)

In 2020, the main primary diseases of recipients demanding lung transplant were idiopathic pulmonary fibrosis (IPF), chronic obstructive pulmonary disease (COPD), secondary pulmonary interstitial fibrosis and pneumoconiosis, each accounting for 38.2%, 21.8%, 13.1% and 10.1%. In addition, recipients with bronchiectasis, pulmonary hypertension, bronchiolitis obliterans syndrome (BOS), lymphangioleiomyomatosis (LAM) and transplant lung failure accounted for 5.7%, 3.1%, 1.5%, 1.4% and 1.1% respectively (Figure 6–5).

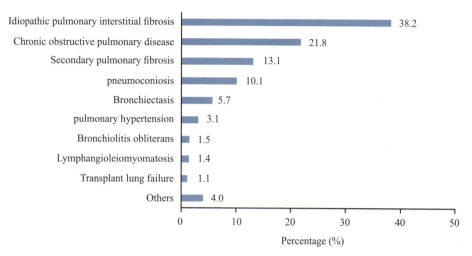

▲ **Figure 6-5** **Distribution of primary diseases of lung transplant recipients in China in 2020 (not including Hong Kong, Macao, and Taiwan regions)**

6.3 Quality analysis of lung transplantation

6.3.1 Operation methods

In 2020, single lung and double lung transplant accounted for 37.2 % and 62.8% respectively. 15% of lung transplants occurred in the emergency department. The percentage of usage of Extracorporeal Membrane Oxygenation (ECMO) during the operation was 68.7%.

6.3.2 Blood transfusion during operation

Median blood transfusion volume during lung transplant operation was 1012.5 (IQR 520.0~1840.0)ml. The proportions of blood transfusion volume ＜500ml, 500~999ml, 1000~1499ml, 1500~1999ml and ≥2000ml were 24.2%, 20.3%, 20.3%, 11.6%, and 23.6%, respectively.

6.3.3 Early (less than 30 days) postoperative complications

Major early postoperative complications were infection (64.6%), renal insufficiency (29.4%), primary lung graft dysfunction (13.2%), tracheal anastomotic lesions (10.3%) and acute rejection (5.9%) (Figure 6-6).

6.3.4 Status at discharge

In 2020, the median length-of-stay of lung transplant recipients in China was 31.0 days (IQR 17.0~51.0). Their perioperative survival rate was 83.5%. Causes of death of lung transplant recipients during the perioperative period were mainly shock or respiratory and circulatory failure caused by lung infection (41.3%), multiple organ failure (30.7%), sudden cardiac death (8.0%), and hemorrhagic shock (5.3%) (Figure 6-7).

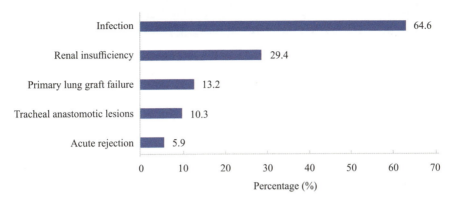

▲ **Figure 6−6** **Perioperative period conditions of lung transplant recipients in 2020 (not including Hong Kong, Macao, and Taiwan regions)**

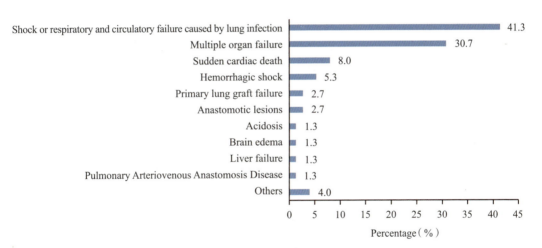

▲ **Figure 6−7** **Cause of death of lung transplant recipients during the perioperative period in 2020 (not including Hong Kong, Macao, and Taiwan regions)**

6.3.5 Postoperative survival

The postoperative (< 30 days), 3−month, 6−month, 1−year and 3−year survival rates of double-lung transplant recipients were 80.5%, 69.9%, 66.6%, 62.7%, and 54.1% respectively. The numbers for single-lung transplant recipients were 83.9%, 76.8%, 72.1%, 65.8% and 54.0% respectively. The single-lung transplant recipients have a higher short-term survival rate than the double-lung transplant recipients (Table 6−2).

6.4 Features and prospects

In recent years, the National Quality Control Center for Lung Transplantation has been continuously improving the clinical diagnosis and treatment system for lung transplantation and has

Table 6-2 Postoperative survival rates of lung transplant recipients in Mainland China (not including Hong Kong, Macao, and Taiwan regions)

	Perioperative period (< 30 day)	3-month	6-month	1-year	3-year
Double lung (%)	80.5	69.9	66.6	62.7	54.1
Single lung (%)	83.9	76.8	72.1	65.8	54.0

been devoted to promoting standardized lung transplantation techniques. Lung transplantation in China in 2020 has continued the trend of increasing from 2019. In 2020, major breakthroughs have been made in the field of lung transplantation for severe COVID-19 patients. At the meantime, rate of postoperative complications, including acute lung transplantation, postoperative infection, primary graft dysfunction, sudden cardiac death and renal insufficiency, etc., remained at a relatively high level.

During the outbreak of COVID-19, China performed the first double-lung transplant for a patient with end-stage COVID-19 related respiratory failure in the world, published the operation principle regarding 'highly selective, high-level protection COVID-19–related lung transplantation, providing the Chinese experience on the treatment of end-stage COVID-19 respiratory failure patients to the whole world.

Emergency lung transplant patients are usually with critical conditions, and the operation time is often very limited. These patients are at higher risks during operation, with higher postoperative rejection rates, higher primary graft dysfunction rates, and lower perioperative and lower long-term survival rates. Therefore, we should promote the establishment of pre-operative evaluation systems to monitor the recipients' transplant contraindications and indications in a strict manner.

As for infection control, we should continue to promote the construction of a whole-process, multi-step infection control mechanism, implementing prevention and control of infection from multiple levels including preoperative evaluation, donor quality maintenance, surgical operation, and postoperative management. For the prevention and treatment of primary graft failure, the quality of the donor should be fully controlled. For recipients with poor physical condition, the use of *ex vivo* circulatory assistance techniques or the appropriate extension of application time of ECMO should be taken into consideration. For the prevention and treatment of sudden cardiac death, transplant team should pay attention to the preoperative assessment of the recipient's cardiac function. Dynamic monitoring of cardiac function during the postoperative period is also essential to help deal with abnormal cardiac symptoms. For the prevention and treatment of renal insufficiency, attention should be paid to the monitoring of drug dosage and renal function indicators. Drug-drug interactions should be given special caution to avoid increased burden on kidneys.

Compared to other countries, lung transplant recipients in China are with higher age and more severe primary diseases. There are more patients with pulmonary fibrosis demanding lung transplant in China, and surgeries are more difficult to perform. Ventilator usage time and median cold ischemia time of donor lungs are also longer than the international averages. These are all reasons for the lower survival rate in China compared with that reported by the International Society for Heart and Lung Transplantation (ISHLT). In the future, we are going to strengthen the monitoring on quality of lung transplants according to the revised quality control indicators on the clinical application of lung transplant techniques. By continuously improving the procedures and technical standards, as well as forming multi-disciplinary lung transplant teams, we believe that the quality of lung transplants in China will be constantly enhanced.

Chapter 7 Technology development and innovation of organ transplantation in China

7.1 Ischemia-free organ transplantation (IFOT)

Under the traditional organ transplantation procedure, the blood flow of organ is blocked for a long time. Ischemia reperfusion injury (IRI), the main factors affecting transplant efficacy and organ utilization, is inevitable during procurement, preservation and implantation, which can cause serious complications, including non-functioning primary grafts and early graft dysfunction. After eight years of exploration, Professor He Xiaoshun's team has developed the first Multi-visceral Support System (Life-X). This machine can create perfusion pressure, temperature, oxygenation and nutritional support for organs *ex vivo*, creating an environment close to the physiological state for the organs, thus maintaining the organ vitality *ex vivo* for a long time and repair damaged organs. Based on this Multi-visceral Support System, the transplant team led by Professor He Xiaoshun created a new procedure of organ transplantation to avoid the blockage of blood flow. The first case of ischemia-free organ transplantation in human using this technique was completed in 2017. Upon completion, there was no IRI in the transplanted liver, such as apoptosis, release of inflammatory factors, or activation of injury pathways. Compared to the traditional technique, the postoperative aspartate aminotransferase (AST) was reduced by 74.7%; alanine aminotransferase ALT was decreased by 77.7%; the primary non-function decreased from 3.1% to 0%; the early allograft dysfunction decreased from 50.0% to 5.3%; the post-reflow syndrome decreased from 81.8% to 6.5%; ICU stay time was shortened from 43.5 hours to 34 hours; and the one-year survival rate increased by 9.8%. Since the organs obtain a normal blood supply and temperature throughout the transplant process, the injuries to the functions of important organs such as the heart, lungs and kidneys by the low temperature in the traditional "cold transplantation" were avoided, and the risk of surgery is greatly reduced. After the success of IFOT, the team carried out the world's first ischemia-free kidney transplantation in 2018.

7.2 Auto liver transplantation in China

The first auto liver transplantation was reported by Professor Pichlmayr in 1989. In China, Professor Huang Jiefu has initially used ALT (Auto liver transplantation, ALT) technology to treat echinococcosis in 2005. While less than 200 cases of ALT have been performed overseas, the Chinese experts have performed more than 300 ALT, which formed the largest case group globally. Leading experts include Academician Dong Jiahong, Academician Zheng Shusen, Professor Ye Qifa, Professor Wen Hao and the team of West China Hospital, Sichuan University. Auto liver transplantation is the application of liver transplantation to the space-occupying lesions in the liver that cannot be resected by conventional surgical procedures. With liver perfusion and venous bypass, surgeons remove liver lesions in *ex vivo* orante-situm way. After repairing and preservation, the recovered liver will be implanted *in situ*, making a radical treatment of hepatic space-occupying lesions. The ALT provides the possibility of surgical treatment for benign or malignant liver-occupied lesions or severe liver trauma that cannot be surgically treated with conventional methods. Compared with allogeneic liver transplantation, this technique does not require allogeneic livers nor immunosuppressant, thus reduces drug costs and associated complications and produces important social and economic benefits. Professor Ye Qifa's team has formulated technical specifications of ALT preoperative liver function evaluation, calculation of liver resection rate, intraoperative perfusion technology and preservation method, as well as function maintenance of preserved livers. These specifications have become an international consensus, and played a key role in promoting the ALT technology.

7.3 Precision treatment of immunosuppressive agents for organ transplantation

The application of calcineurin (CNIs) tacrolimus has greatly reduced rejection after transplantation and improved the survival rate of transplanted organs. However, as CNIs has a narrow therapeutic window, significant differences in pharmacokinetic parameters between individuals and the appropriate dosage for different individuals varies a lot. Therefore, "tailored" accurate diagnosis and treatment plan of CNIs is urgently needed. Studies have shown that the gene polymorphism of drug metabolism enzyme CYP3A5 is the main reason for the tacrolimus concentration differences in plasma of patients. There is a 6986A>G mutation (RS776746, CYP3A5*3) in the 3rd intron of *CYP3A5* gene at position 22893. This SNP can lead to abnormal splicing of CYP3A5 mRNA and lead to premature cleavage of CYP3A5 protein by the stop codon, thus causing the loss of enzyme activity. The expression and activity of CYP3A5 protein in liver and intestine were significantly decreased in CYP3A5*3 homozygous individuals. Activity of enzyme decline leads to elevated tacrolimus blood concentration level. The Alliance of the Implementation of Clinical Pharmacogenomics Guidelines recommend that transplant recipients with CYP3A5*3 genotype should reduce the dosage of tacrolimus to avoid adverse drug reactions.

Since 2008, Professor Ye Qifa from the National Health Committee Transplantation Medicine Engineering Technology Center, jointly with and academician of Chinese Academy of Engineering, Academician Zhou Honghao, leading the transplant teams from Zhongnan Hospital of Wuhan University and The Third Xiangya Hospital of Central South University, have started their research on recommending the different initial dose of tacrolimus according to different genotypes. Sanger sequencing method was used to detect the *CYP3A5* genotype of patients before transplantation. At present, more than 2120 cases have been completed, and the mutation frequency of CYP3A5*3 homozygous individuals was found to be as high as 52.90%, suggesting that dose of tacrolimus should be reduced by 50% in more than half of the detected population. After giving the corresponding initial dose according to the genotype, the patient's tacrolimus concentration compliance rate increased from 37.5% to 77.8% within 7 days, and the proportion of tacrolimus dosage needing adjustment decreased from 55.6% to 22.3%. The rate of rejection and adverse drug poisoning reaction dropped significantly within 3 months. Among the recommended initial dosage group, tacrolimus cost was significantly lower in the fast-metabolized group than in the control group within 7 days after transplantation. Tacrolimus drug does was significantly higher in the slow metabolic group than in the control group. At the meantime, the cost of rejection treatment was significantly reduced in both groups.

At present, this technology has been popularized and applied in transplant centers nationwide, and a precise, rapid, efficient, convenient and economical detection kit for CYP3A5*3 gene polymorphism has been developed, which will play a positive role in promoting the fulfillment of clinical individualized treatment of CNIs drugs and improving the transplant prognosis.

7.4 New technique of vena cava and right atrium anastomosis liver transplantation (VC-AALT)

Vana Cava and atrium anastomotic liver transplantation (VC-AALT) was initiated by Professor Ye Qifa's team in 1996. It is used for the treatment of Budd-Chiari syndrome (BCS) and has shown great effect on preventing the recurrence of BCS.

The core of this technology is to preserve or resect the retrohepatic inferior vena cava, or resect the suprahepatic vena cava, or ligate the suprahepatic vena cava under the atrium, or complete the resection of the retrohepatic inferior vena cava and the sick liver under ECMO bypass (tumor spreading atrium), in accordance with the different lesions of the inferior vena cava. Then, the anastomosis of the suprahepatic vena cava of the donor liver and the side of the right atrium is completed. The infrahepatic vena cava of the donor liver is anastomosed with the recipient inferior vena cava.

A single transplantation center has performed over 30 cases of VC-AALT. The long-term follow-up study has showed that the 1-year, 3-year and 5-year survival rates were 88.89%, 83.33% and 77.78% respectively. Compared with the first 4 cases reported abroad in 2018, China's experience is 22 years ahead of the rest of the world. Based on the varying pathological progression of BCS, Professor Ye Qifa's team has created the bridge-piggyback liver transplantation (B-PBLT), atrial suspension liver transplantation (ASLT), vena cava resection bridge liver transplantation (VCRBLT), ECMO bypass VC-AALT, and auxiliary para-lateral atrial suspension liver transplantation.

The application of VC-AALT in BCS has greatly prevented the recurrence of BCS (BCS often recurs after conventional liver transplantation and piggyback liver transplantation, because posterior vena cava, suprahepatic vena cava, and hepatic venous lesions cannot be removed with the conventional methods), provided new technique for the treatment of end-stage liver cirrhosis, liver cancer merger posterior hepatic vena cava sponge lesion, vena cava occlusion, vena cava thrombus and diseases such as tumor spread to the right atrium. It also opened a new way of treatment for patients with childhood metabolic disease, orthotopic auxiliary liver transplantation, and patients with difficult on reconstruction of venous return.

7.5 Split Liver Transplantation (SLT)

7.5.1 Introduction to Split Liver Transplantation (SLT)

Donor liver sources have been expanded by the use of marginal donor livers, living-related livers, donation after cardiac death (DCD), etc. However, the issue of liver shortage has not been tackled, thus constrained the development of liver transplant in China. In 1984, Brismuth et al. reported the first reduced-sized orthotopic liver graft in hepatic transplantation in children, liver transplantation with a reduced-sized graft has been a golden standard for pediatric liver transplantation ever since. The thinking of one liver with dual purpose has become clear. In 1988, Pichlmayr et al. pioneered the first split liver transplantation (SLT) in the world, enabling the transplantation of one donor liver into two recipients – one pediatric and one adult patient. In the same year, Brismuth et al. performed the first SLT with one donor liver transplanted to 2 adult recipients. Compared to living donor liver transplantation (LDLT), the source of SLT is cadaveric donation. SLT has higher requirements for the surgical technique of liver transplantation, but it does not cause surgical risks to the donor, and dual-purpose liver use could help allocate donor livers in a more reasonable way. In the early stage of SLT, the postoperative prognosis of patients in various transplant centers in the world was not good enough. The survival rate and rate of complications also varied from each site. Furthermore, rate of biliary complications after SLT was significantly higher than those of whole liver transplantation, which could be up to 40% in the early phase. However, as the formulation of consensus regarding donor-recipient matching and vascular allocation principles among centers, and the maturing of SLT related techniques, survival rates of STL in different centers have been improving gradually. As for now, the 1–year survival rate has reached 80%~90%, rates of blood vessels bile ducts related complications have also decreased significantly.

7.5.2 SLT in China

China has entered the era of organ donation from citizens after death since 2015. Shortage of donor livers has also become a motivation for transplant centers of developing SLT related techniques. Statistics show that the cases of SLT performed in Mainland China in 2015 and 2016 were 34 and 41, respectively. The number has been increasing ever since. 140 cases were performed in 2018, more than 200 cases were performed in 2019, and 387 cases were performed in 2020. A total of 964 cases of SLT have been performed from 2015 to 2020. Transplant centers that performed most cases of SLT were: Renji Hospital, School of Medicine, Shanghai Jiaotong University (172); Tianjin First Central Hospital (167); the Third Hospital Affiliated to the Sun Yat-Sen University (133); the First Affiliated Hospital, Zhejiang University School of Medicine (116) and the West China Hospital, Sichuan University (67). In addition, it is worth noting that from 2018 to 2020, the number of SLT recipients under the age of 18 was 81, 139, and 197, respectively, which exceeded 50% of the total number of recipients, indicating that minors are still the main targets of SLT.

According to different procuring methods, SLT can be divided into two types: *in-vivo* SLT and *ex-vivo* SLT. During *in-vivo* SLT, the blood flow of the donor liver will not be cut off, thus cold ischemia time could be significantly reduced. At the same time, *in-vivo* SLT could help identify the hepatic artery, hepatic vein, bile duct and other tissues, thus reduce rates of complications including hepatic cross-section hemorrhage and biliary fistula, etc., and help realize more reasonable allocation of donor liver blood vessels. With all the above advantages, *in-vivo* SLT has been widely adopted by the international community.

Conventional liver splitting methods include the classic splitting method and the complete left & right hemi-liver splitting methods. Classic splitting refers to splitting the donor liver into the left lateral lobe (II~ III) and the extended right trilobe (I & IV~ VIII), which is mainly used when the recipents are a combination of child and adult. Splitting the donor liver into the left hemiliver (segments I to IV) and the right hemiliver (segments V to VIII) is called complete left and right hepatic splitting, which is used for 2 adult recipients with matching weights. For this kind of surgeries, the distribution of the middle hepatic vein should strictly follow the direction of the middle hepatic vein, anatomical characteristics, and volume of left and right livers. Academician Zheng Shusen and his team from the First Affiliated Hospital of Zhejiang University, School of Medicine, used cold-stored iliac vein allografts to bridge the hepatic venous outflow tract, and maintained the hepatic vein reflux of the V and VIII segments, making the right hepatic living donor liver transplantation without middle hepatic vein and SLT a safe and reliable operation methods.

In addition to the increasing improvement of surgical methods, understanding of the principles of donor and recipient evaluation and matching has also been enhanced within the Chinese transplant community. In October, 2020, the first Experts Consensus on Split Liver Transplantation was published by the Surgery Branch of Chinese Medical Association, which promoted the standardization and normalization of SLT in China. Research has indicated that split-liver transplants have similar prognosis to whole-liver grafts, while the former has more strict selection criteria for donors and recipients. SLT surgeries are usually limited to donor livers with ideal conditions in liver volume, liver function, age, blood circulation, etc. At present, the donor liver standards followed by Chinese experts include: (a) donor is younger than 50–years-old; (b) liver function is basically normal, with no or only mild fatty liver (< 10%); (c) the hemodynamic indicators are stable, the donor does not need support from a large dose of vasoactive drugs; (d) ICU admission time is less than 5 days; (e) serum sodium is less than 160 mmol/L, etc.

7.5.3 Summary

Since 2015, China has fully entered the era of livers from organ donation after the death of citizens, while the issue of donor liver shortage is still severe. SLT, as a mature method of liver transplantation, can effectively expand the source of donor livers and shorten the waiting time for recipients. Through careful assessment of donors and recipients and skilled SLT surgical techniques, the postoperative efficacy of SLT can be significantly improved. Under a reasonable organ allocation policy and multi-center cooperation, China will promote the development of SLT in a safe and standard manner to better serve the people.

7.6 The clinical treatment of adult kidney transplantation with pediatric-donor kidney from low-age, low-weight infants and toddlers has been continuously improved, well clinical outcomes have been achieved

Organ donation rates in China is lower than that of the developed countries. The relative lack of donated organs is still a long-term problem. Compared with adults, pediatric donation is relatively easy to expand because their social relations are relatively simple, and their parents or other legal guardians are more likely to accept the concept of organ donation. Therefore, children and even infants' organ donation can expand the donor pool and deserve further attention. Adult kidney transplantation with infant donor kidney generally adopts *en bloc* double kidney transplantation. Due to the difficulty of the operation, vascular and ureteral complications are prone to occur post transplantation. The first case was reported in the 1970s internationally, while the first case in China was reported in 1981. However, reports of this type of transplantation were rare in the following 30 years. With the progress of the system construction of organ donation from Chinese citizens after death, as well as the continuous improvement of surgical technology, innovative progress has been made to overcome the risk of anesthesia during operation, improved the donor and recipient vascular anastomosis, as well as accurately handled the contradiction between anticoagulation-bleeding after operation. These innovations contribute a lot to the prevention and treatment of postoperative complications. Hence in recent years, more hospitals started to perform the *en bloc* kidney transplantation for newborns donor with low body weight (< 5kg), or other children of low age. Although the number of cases is still low, existing experiences have showed promising outcomes. Union Hospital affiliated to Tongji Medical College of Huazhong University of Science and Technology retrospectively analyzed 38 *en-bloc* kidney transplants and found that the one-year graft survival rate was 76.3% and the recipient survival rate was 100.0%. The study was published in the *Chinese Journal of Organ Transplantation* in 2021.

7.7 Application of metagenomics next-generation sequencing in the diagnosis and treatment of pulmonary infection after renal transplantation

Pulmonary infection is the most common cause of post-operative infection and death in the recipients of kidney transplantation. Particularly, mortality rate of multi-pathogen mixed infection can reach 50%. Rapid identification of pathogenic microorganisms is the key to treatment. Conventional ways of detection, including bacterial cultivation, gram staining, immunoassay and nucleic acid detection, etc., are usually with relatively low timeliness, sensitivity, and specificity, not meeting the need of the early diagnosis and treatment of severe infection.

Metagenomic next-generation sequencing (mNGS) is a new pathogenic microorganism identification method, which has experienced rapid development in the past 5 years. Through high-throughput sequencing of nucleic acid in clinical samples, this technology can quickly and objectively detect a variety of pathogenic microorganisms (including viruses, bacteria, fungi, parasites, etc.), and is especially suitable for the primary diagnosis of acute, critical and difficult infections. As mNGS has the advantages of fast detection, high accuracy, wide coverage and less influence of antibiotics on test results, some large domestic medical institutions have additionally applied the mNGS in the diagnosis and treatment of severe inflammation after kidney transplantation other than routine examinations in recent years. The mNGS can determine the pathogen of pulmonary infection within 24–48 hours, adding great diagnostic value for severe pneumonia caused by mixed infection, pneumocystis and cytomegalovirus infection after kidney transplantation. This technology is also helpful to guide the clinical application of antibiotics and help improve the prognosis. Related studies have been published in *Ann Transplant* and *Bioengineered*, etc., in 2021.

7.8 Optimization of perioperative management strategies for heart transplantation

Heart transplantation is the most effective treatment for patients with end-stage heart failure. The key points for tackling the problem brought by the contradiction between the huge heart failure population and the scarce donor resources are standardizing the treatment for heart failure disease patients, optimizing the normalized evaluation, and selection for heart transplant recipients, etc.

The constantly standardizing treatment for heart failure has delayed the progression of heart failure patients. Therefore, we could provide the limited donor resources to the heart failure patients who were urgent and can benefit most to fulfill maximum utilization of the donor resources.

In regards to perioperative management, most transplant centers have established multidisciplinary heart failure and heart transplantation treatment teams. Some of them have explored and developed the best strategies of different mechanical circulation support as a bridge to heart transplantation, performed the largest number of heart transplantation undergoing mechanical circulation support (including ECMO, IABP and ECMO combining IABP and left ventricular assist device) in China, and established the evaluation and perioperative management strategies for recipients with pulmonary hypertension before transplantation. These accomplishments reduced the mortality rate of critical recipients during waiting period and perioperative mortality of heart transplantation, thus greatly improved the short-term and long-term survival of heart transplant patients.

7.9 Independent development and clinical application of artificial heart

In terms of alternative treatment for heart transplantation, China has developed three third-generation all-magnetic levitation artificial hearts with independent intellectual property rights. Multiple-center clinical trials are being performed currently. These third-generation artificial hearts adopt magnetic levitation non-contact bearing, are with small size and good biocompatibility, featuring the most advanced technology in the world. At present, 25 clinical trials have been completed in Fuwai Hospital of Chinese Academy of Medical Sciences and Union Hospital of Tongji Medical College of Huazhong University of Science and Technology.

7.10 Lobar transplantation with the split lung technique

For patients with small thoracic cavity or children, it is extremely difficult to wait for a donor lung of an appropriate size. Lobar transplantation with the split lung technique can solve this problem. Moreover, the postoperative effect has no significant difference from that of normal lung transplantation. In the past, in the split right lung transplantation, lungs are usually split into upper, middle and lower lobar. While the upper and lower lobar were transplanted to two patients respectively, the middle lobar was often discarded to avoid the presence of the middle tracheal stump. The lung transplantation team of Wuxi People's Hospital performed the world's first split right upper/middle lobe and right lower lobe transplantation, where they rebuilt and generated the right upper/middle lobe tracheal opening cuff to be anastomosed. This procedure preserves the right middle lobe and increases the patient's postoperative lung volume. On the other hand, shortening the middle segment of the trachea can reduce the useless cavity of the right lower lung, which is helpful for airway anastomosis and repair. The results of tracheoscopy and chest imaging showed a good lung dilatation and no obvious anastomotic complications. This procedure proved the strategy safe and feasible. As a special kind of lung lobe transplantation, it is worthy to popularize in centers with adequate experience. A detailed case report, "*A Modified Lobar Technique Combining RUL and RML for Small therapy*", was published in The *Annals of Thoracic Surgery*.

7.11 Heterotopic lung transplantation

The development of lung transplantation in recent years has been constrained by donor shortage. The outbreak of COVID-19 pandemic has further exacerbated the issue. With the development of lung transplantation tracheal anastomosis, heterotopic lung transplantation has broken through the shackles of conventional methods, allowing the lungs that could only be given up to be reused to save the lives of critically ill patients. The lung transplantation team of Wuxi People's Hospital has performed a total of 4 cases of heterotopic lung transplantation, including 3 cases of single heterotopic lung transplantation (1 case of left donor lung transplantation to the right chest, 2 cases of right donor lung transplantation to the left chest). In the three patients, one donor lung was rotated 180° along the vertical axis and then implanted into the contralateral thoracic cavity. The membrane and cartilage of the donor bronchus and the recipient bronchus were staggered and anastomosed. The pulmonary artery of the donor was fully freed along the pulmonary artery trunk. The length is sufficient to extend to the front side of the bronchial axis to be anastomosed with the recipient's pulmonary artery to ensure that there is no tension during the anastomosis. The pulmonary vein atrial sleeve was anastomosed using the conventional method. The other case was a split bilateral lobe heterotopic transplantation in a female patient with a small chest cavity. The right lung of the donor was split anatomically into the right upper lung and the right middle and lower lung. The upper right lung is rotated and implanted into the left thoracic cavity of the recipient and the right middle and lower lung is implanted into the right thoracic cavity. All operations were successfully completed; during follow-up, the recipient's bronchoscopy and chest imaging results showed that the transplanted lung was well expanded and morphologically able to adapt and fill the chest cavity over time, proving the safety and feasibility of heterotopic lung transplantation.

7.12 Combined heart-lung transplants

For patients with end-stage cardiopulmonary failure, combined heart-lung transplant is the only effective treatment. The limited development of combined heart-lung transplant is mainly due to the high surgical difficulty and serious complications, especially posterior mediastinal hemorrhage. The lung transplantation team of the First Affiliated Hospital of Guangzhou Medical University has made great efforts and technical improvements to address this prominent problem, and innovatively developed the micro-heterotopic combined heart-lung transplant. Traditional combined heart-lung transplantation requires the removal of the carina of the recipient and the left and right main bronchus, and then the trachea of the donor and recipient are anastomosed in situ. Micro-heterotopic cardiopulmonary transplantation is to cut off the recipient's trachea, no longer removing the carina and left and right main bronchus, but remain in the recipient's body after intracavitary treatment and stack the donor trachea on the recipient's carina. The convexity is anastomosed with the proximal end of the trachea of the recipient. This method reduces the scope of posterior mediastinal resection, reduces surgical bleeding, especially for those with abundant collateral circulation, and shortens the operation time. The technical article *"Non-In Situ Technology of Heart-Lung Transplantation: Case Series and Technique Description"* was published in the *Annals of Thoracic Surgery*.

7.13 Innovative method for potential organ donor evaluation

According to the current situation of organ donation in China, with the purpose of facilitating the timely identification, assessment and reporting of potential organ donors by medical staff in all types of hospitals at all levels, especially primary healthcare settings, the OPO of the General Hospital of Southern Theatre Command (GHOPO) innovatively proposed a convenient method for potential organ donor evaluation-ABC-HOME. The method classified candidates by Age, irreversible Brain damage or Brain death, Contradiction and Circulation situation as "ABC". Those who meet the ABC standards could be identified as possible donors. In addition, the method describes History (clinical history), Organ function, Medication history and internal Environment as "HOME". Patients meeting the ABD-HOME criteria could be identified as potential donors. On this basis, after gaining informed consent from the family member, the potential donors could be converted to actual donors. The application of ABC-HOME method significantly improved the reporting rate of potential organ donors, and significantly increased the number of potential organ donors generated per ICU bed.